Networks of Innovation offers an historical perspective on the manner in which private-sector organizations have acquired, sustained, and periodically lost the ability to develop, manufacture, and market new serum antitoxins and vaccines. The primary focus is on the H. K. Mulford Co., on Sharp & Dohme, which acquired Mulford in 1929, and upon Merck & Co., Inc., which merged with Sharp & Dohme in 1953. By surveying a century of innovation in biologicals, the authors are able to analyze the conditions that either promoted or prevented creative changes in this important industry. They show how the activities of these three commercial enterprises were related to a series of complex networks of scientific, governmental, and medical institutions in the United States and abroad. This is the first such history to draw extensively on sources internal to Merck, one of the world's leading innovators in modern vaccines and pharmaceuticals.

NETWORKS OF INNOVATION

NETWORKS OF INNOVATION

Vaccine Development at
Merck, Sharp & Dohme, and Mulford, 1895–1995

LOUIS GALAMBOS WITH JANE ELIOT SEWELL

The Johns Hopkins University

and

The Business History Group

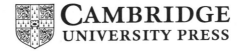

CAMBRIDGE
UNIVERSITY PRESS

PUBLISHED BY THE PRESS SYNDICATE OF THE UNIVERSITY OF CAMBRIDGE
The Pitt Building, Trumpington Street, Cambridge CB2 1RP

CAMBRIDGE UNIVERSITY PRESS
The Edinburgh Building, Cambridge CB2 2RU, United Kingdom
40 West 20th Street, New York, NY 10011-4211, USA
10 Stamford Road, Oakleigh, Melbourne 3166, Australia

First published 1995
First paperback edition 1997

Printed in the United States of America

Library of Congress Cataloging-in-Publication Data

Galambos, Louis.
Networks of innovation : vaccine development at Merck, Sharp & Dohme,
and Mulford, 1895-1995 / Louis Galambos, Jane Eliot Sewell.
p.   cm.
ISBN 0-521-56308-9 (hc)
1. Vaccines – History. 2. Vaccines industry – History. 3. Merck, Sharp & Dohme
International – History. I. Sewell, Jane Eliot. II. Title.
RM281.G35   1995   95-42794
615'.372 –dc20   CIP

A catalog record for this book is available from the British Library.

ISBN 0-521-56308-9 hardback
ISBN 0-521-62620-X paperback

The following trademarks, which appear in type form different from that of surrounding text, are trademarks used in connection with current or past products of Merck & Co., Inc.: *S.T. 37, Purivax, Rubeovax, Gammagee, Dryvax, Attenuvax, Mumpsvax, Meruvax, M-M-R, M-M-Vax, M-R-Vax, Biavax, DEPTAVAC-HVT, Adjuvant 65, Timoptic, Clinoril, Mefoxin, Meningovax-C, Meningovax A/C, Pneumovax, Pneumovax 23, PedvaxHIB, HEP-B-GAMMAGEE, Heptavax-B, Recombivax HB, Mectizan, Vasotec, Primaxin, Mevacor, M-M-R II, Varivax, Vaqta, S.Q., Nicrazin, Amprol, Hepzide, Thibenzole, Dolobid, Fluax.*

To our families

CONTENTS

PREFACE

LL OF THOSE readers who were rendered nervous by Richard Preston's bestseller, *The Hot Zone*,[1] may find comfort in the following account of a century of increasingly successful efforts to develop vaccine and serum antitoxin defenses against infection. They will be comforted, we believe, but not entirely relieved of concern. The search continues. Viruses and bacteria continue to emerge and evolve, posing new threats to human life and health. The quest for preventive medicines has a history with chapters but no conclusion. As long as there is human life, we will need institutions that will sustain the search for innovative means of fighting infection.

In *Networks of Innovation*, our emphasis is on the private sector's contribution to the process of innovation in vaccines and antitoxins. But as our title indicates, we placed the activities of the H. K. Mulford Company, Sharp & Dohme, and Merck & Co., Inc., in their historical context — a context that identifies the complex, loosely integrated institutional and personal networks that fostered innovation in this industry. The first of the networks that we examine took shape in the late nineteenth century around the central ideas of the bacteriological revolution. Other networks with distinctive leaders, values, scientific findings, and organizations followed during the twentieth century. Many

---

1 (New York, 1995).

of the relevant institutions in these networks were nonprofit professional organizations; many of the leaders were scientists in universities and research organizations. There were, as well, public institutions, including a rich array of public health organizations at the local, state, and federal levels in the United States. Other institutions in these networks were international in scope. The mixed system that gradually evolved was unusually creative, and we have described in some detail the contribution to that process of the three companies studied.

We did not select these three firms at random. We launched this project by writing for Merck & Co., Inc., an internal study of the century of vaccine and serum antitoxin development that took place at Mulford (which Sharp & Dohme acquired in 1929), at Sharp & Dohme (which merged with Merck in 1953), and at the parent company – one of the four leading vaccine firms in the world today. Then, with the active support of Dr. R. Gordon Douglas, Jr., and Merck Vaccines, we did the additional research, analysis, and writing necessary to convert the study into a scholarly account for the Cambridge University Press. To some considerable extent, our focus shifted from Merck and its predecessor organizations to the complex network of individuals and institutions that sustained – and sometimes impeded – innovation in biologicals. To its credit, Merck gave us complete freedom of interpretation, limited only by the necessity to be factually accurate about the science and medicine of vaccines and antitoxins.

In our effort to historicize the private sector, we have focused on the ability of companies to develop scientific and technological capabilities. In that regard, this book is a business history that builds on the pioneering work Alfred D. Chandler has done on organizational capabilities. It is a business history with a twist provided by the scholars in economics and business policy who have of late logged significant advances in the analysis of organizational capabilities. We have added to this scholarship histories and analyses of three organizations: one of which developed new capabilities *ab ovo*; another of which was unable to do so; and a third of which created an organization capable of sustaining innovation in science and technology over the long term. This third company, Merck & Co., Inc., weathered the struggles of the 1970s, the transition to a new long cycle of scientific/technological development in the 1980s, and a bruising confrontation with the Clinton Administration in the 1990s. By examining a full century of innovation at these three organizations, we hope to provide an historical perspective that much of the current work in business policy and economics lacks.

As should be clear, our book is also a study in the history of medicine. Scholars in this field have written very little about the role of private pharmaceutical and biological firms in the development of preventive medicines. We know substantially more about public health contributions to immunization than we do about the companies that have developed, produced, and distributed the bulk of the vaccines and antitoxins used in the United States. We hope that *Networks of Innovation* will encourage other scholars to analyze the history of companies in this industry and to bring into historical focus the intricate relationships that have emerged between nonprofit, public, and profit-making institutions in this country and abroad.

By focusing upon innovation in a science-based industry, we have also positioned this book on the edge of the social history of science and close to the center of the history of technology. In both subdisciplines, there is an interest in change, in the interaction of ideas, individuals, and institutions. Both deal with historical processes that have been central to the evolution of modern societies. We have followed that lead, staking out for examination a specific trail through a century of rapid transformation in medical science and biotechnology. While our research was specific to the industry, the organizations, and the networks studied, we believe those historical episodes suggest some general conclusions about the ability of organizations to adjust to changes in their environments and to shape their futures in creative ways.

We also touch upon political history, especially in our treatment of the regulatory environment in the United States and the various immunization programs introduced following World War II.

From the perspective of these three firms, we follow the development in the United States of a mixed system of political economy in biologicals. This system continued to change over the one hundred years we have examined and it is still changing today. Many of these transformations encouraged innovation. Others did not. On balance, however, America's mixed system of professional, public, and commercial institutions appears over the long term to have done an excellent job of generating new antitoxins and vaccines. Certainly the U.S. historical record in this regard is more favorable than its performance in ensuring high levels of immunization. We discuss the latter problem when we consider the Clinton Administration's recent effort to transform the political economy of vaccines.

In our research for *Networks of Innovation*, we have been able to draw upon many sources internal to these three firms. Although we could not always locate specific sources we wanted, the archival record that has survived enabled us to offer more of an internal view of the process of innovation than has heretofore been available to scholars. If readers agree, then we all have Merck & Co., Inc., Gordon Douglas, and Merck Vaccines to thank for this unusual opportunity to place in historical perspective a century of innovation in antitoxins and vaccines.

CHAPTER 1

1894: "THE FOREMOST MEDICAL QUESTION OF THE DAY"

I N 1894, many Americans were deeply concerned about labor violence, about an economy sliding into the worst depression the country had ever experienced, and about the adverse impact mass immigration seemed to be having on urban life. To many middle-class Americans, the new immigrants from southern Europe were especially troublesome. Crowded into slums, living in tenements, the immigrants were associated by the "better" class of citizens with corrupt ward-level politics, with a breakdown in the country's traditional values, and with urban diseases.[1]

While there was no justification for a moralistic allocation of blame for disease, there was abundant justification for the concerns of the urban middle class. Mortality rates were high for several infectious diseases and the living conditions among recent immigrants in the cities contributed to the incidence of tuberculosis, pneumonia, and diphtheria, three of the leading causes of death in the United States. Physicians had not been able to provide effective therapies for these or other infectious diseases and the morbidity rates were appalling.[2]

---

1 Alan M. Kraut, *Silent Travelers: Germs, Genes, and the "Immigrant Menace"* (Baltimore, 1994), especially pp. 1–9, 50–77, 105–65.

2 Samuel H. Preston and Michael R. Haines, *Fatal Years: Child Mortality in Late Nineteenth-Century America* (Princeton, NJ, 1991). George Rosen, *Preventive Medicine in the United States, 1900–1975: Trends and Interpretations* (New York, 1975),

Concern about these health-related aspects of what was often called "*The* Social Problem" had led to a significant public health movement in this country. In the largest cities, municipal health agencies had struggled for many years to deal with problems of sanitation and sickness. In New York City, a Metropolitan Board of Health had been active since 1866, and after the bacteriological basis of infection began to be understood, the New York Board had established a new Division of Pathology, Bacteriology, and Disinfection to conduct scientific research on infectious diseases. Other cities were launching similar efforts, and during the 1890s, a network of innovative public institutions began to take shape.[3] This network included the bacteriological laboratory of the federal government's Marine Hospital Service.[4]

---

pp. 3–13. Harry F. Dowling, *Fighting Infection: Conquests of the Twentieth Century* (Cambridge, MA, 1977), pp. 228–49.

3 John Duffy, *A History of Public Health in New York City, 1866–1966* (New York, 1974), pp. 1–90. David Blancher, "Workshops of the Bacteriological Revolution: A History of the Laboratories of the New York City Department of Health, 1892–1912" (Ph.D. diss., City University of New York, 1979), pp. 1–2, 20–69. Mazyck P. Ravenel, ed., *A Half Century of Public Health* (New York, 1921), pp. 66–117, 133–96. Barbara Gutmann Rosenkrantz, *Public Health and the State: Changing Views in Massachusetts, 1842–1936* (Cambridge, MA, 1972), pp. 74–127. Judith Walzer Leavitt, *The Healthiest City: Milwaukee and the Politics of Health Reform* (Princeton, NJ, 1982). Stuart Galishoff, *Safeguarding the Public Health: Newark, 1895–1918*, (Westport, CT, 1975), especially pp. 14–43. Fitzhugh Mullan, *Plagues and Politics: The Story of the United States Public Health Service* (New York, 1989), pp. 32–56. H. D. Kramer, "The Germ Theory and the Early Public Health Program in the United States," *Bulletin of the History of Medicine* 22, no. 3 (1948): 233–47.

4 The Marine Hospital Service established its Hygienic Laboratory in 1887 at Staten Island, New York. The lab moved to Washington, D.C., in 1891, and ten years later Congress appropriated a sum to enlarge this "laboratory for the investigation of infectious and contagious diseases and matters pertaining to the public health." The following year, the Marine Hospital Service became the Public Health and Marine Hospital Service. In 1912, Congress dropped "and Marine Hospital" from the name of the Service. Ralph Chester Williams, *The United States Public Health Service, 1798–1950* (Washington, DC, 1951), pp. 166–7, 181.

Many private organizations and individuals established close ties with the emerging public health institutions and contributed to the ability of this loosely integrated network to foster innovation. Physicians and their medical organizations were involved, as were pharmaceutical businesses like the H. K. Mulford Company, "Manufacturing Chemists" of Philadelphia. Mulford produced and distributed various powders, tablets, syrups, tinctures, and antiseptics to pharmacies and physicians. In 1894, the firm's top officers recognized that the public health network[5] was generating some unusual opportunities for private as well as public enterprises and decided to expand their operations to include biological products.[6]

Also see A. Hunter Dupree, *Science in the Federal Government: A History of Policies and Activities to 1940* (Cambridge, MA, 1957), pp. 267–8; J. Parascandola, "The Beginning of Pharmacology in the Federal Government," *Pharmacy in History* 30 (1988): 179–87; and especially Victoria A. Harden, *Inventing the NIH: Federal Biomedical Research Policy, 1887-1937* (Baltimore, 1986), pp. 9–19.

5 For a discussion of the importance of "the ability to access new knowledge from outside the boundaries of the organization" see R. Henderson and I. Cockburn, "Measuring Competence? Exploring Firm Effects in Pharmaceutical Research," *Strategic Management Journal* 15, special issue (1994): 63–84. Alfonso Gambardella, *Science and Innovation: The U.S. Pharmaceutical Industry During the 1980s* (Cambridge, Eng., 1995), uses the idea of networks, but he confines it to specific, contractual relations outside the firm (see especially pp. 146–58). This is the approach taken in the volume of *Research Policy* 20, no. 5 (1991), devoted to "Networks of Innovators" (C. DeBresson and R. Walker, eds.). See also A. Gambardella, "Competitive Advantages from In-House Scientific Research: The U.S. Pharmaceutical Industry in the 1980s," *Research Policy* 21, no. 5 (1992): 391–407. For an analysis of the national "systems" that contain numerous such networks see R. R. Nelson and N. Rosenberg, "Technical Innovation and National Systems," and D. C. Mowery and N. Rosenberg, "The U.S. National Innovation System," both in Richard R. Nelson, ed., *National Innovation Systems: A Comparative Analysis* (New York, 1993), pp. 1–21 and 29–75, respectively.

6 Jonathan Liebenau, *Medical Science and Medical Industry: The Formation of the American Pharmaceutical Industry* (Baltimore, 1987), pp. 58–9; Allan Chase, *Magic Shots: A Human and Scientific Account of the Long and Continuing Struggle to Eradicate Infectious Diseases by Vaccination* (New York, 1982), pp. 180–3.

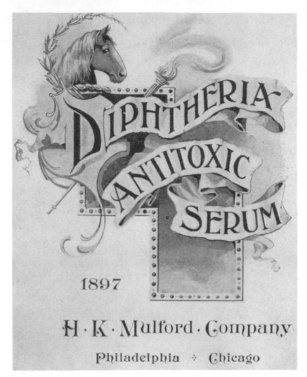

The cover from a Mulford advertising brochure.

The new opportunities in biologicals stemmed from the germ theory experimentation and bacteriology, areas of research that had been the cutting edge of medical science in Europe for the previous thirty years. Fortunately for Mulford, for the American public health institutions, and for the public, Europe exported its ideas as freely as it did the waves of immigrants who were reshaping American urban life. Robert Koch (1843–1910), a German bacteriologist, was the leading scientific innovator in this new field of study. He established the procedures for proving that a particular living agent was the source of a specific disease, for growing single strains of bacteria in pure culture, and for identifying these agents by staining.[7] Louis Pasteur (1822–95),

---

7 These procedures became known universally as "Koch's postulates." *Essays of Robert Koch*, tr. K. Codell Carter (New York, 1987), especially pp. 83–96, 117–27, 129–50.

the distinguished French scientist, was one of the first to apply the principles of bacteriology to the prevention of disease by using the attenuated bacillus of chicken cholera to protect broods against infection (announced in 1880).[8] He also was able to induce immunity against anthrax and rabies in animals and to develop in 1886 a rabies vaccine for human use.[9]

2

These breakthroughs had followed by almost a century the first modern innovation in vaccinology and immunology: Edward Jenner's 1796 development of a safe and effective vaccine for the prevention of smallpox.[10] Jenner was an astute English general practitioner familiar with the ancient and unsafe technique of variolation – the administration of biological matter from smallpox sufferers to create immunity among those who survived the procedure.[11] Using lymph from a patient with the relatively benign disease of cowpox, he successfully vaccinated (the Latin *vaccinus* means "of or pertaining to cows") a young resident of Gloucestershire. Jenner wrote to a friend, "Listen to the most delightful part of my story. The boy has since been inoculated for the smallpox [that is, exposed to the disease] which, as I ventured to predict, pro-

8 W. D. Foster, *A History of Medical Bacteriology and Immunology* (London, 1970). Thomas D. Brock, *Robert Koch: A Life in Medicine and Bacteriology* (Madison, WI, 1988), pp. 94-104, 117–39, 267–85. Koch, *Essays*. René J. Dubos, *Louis Pasteur* (Boston, 1950), pp. 233–330.

9 Dubos, *Pasteur*, pp. 330–43. Chase, *Magic Shots*, pp. 133–8.

10 Jenner performed his successful experiment in 1796; submitted a paper on this subject to the Royal Society in 1797; and after it was rejected, published an extended version as a pamphlet in 1798. On the development of the smallpox vaccine, see Derrick Baxby, *Jenner's Smallpox Vaccine: The Riddle of Vaccinia Virus and Its Origin* (London, 1981); Peter Razzell, *Edward Jenner's Cowpox Vaccine: The History of a Medical Myth* (Sussex, 1977).

11 For a more favorable view of variolation and a description of the 1721–2 Royal Experiment on Immunity ("the first recorded clinical trial in the history of immunity") see Arthur M. Silverstein, *A History of Immunology* (New York, 1989), pp. 24–37.

duced no effect." Jenner had produced immunity to the far more serious disease of smallpox.[12]

The history of smallpox vaccination in the decades that followed is a study in social and intellectual conflict — a pattern of contention that would become a common feature of vaccination programs to the present day. Proponents of variolation argued for the superiority of their technique. Opponents of any public measure to protect the population from disease argued their cases. The result: the disease continued to be a major cause of death, and as late as 1870–5, the western world experienced a smallpox pandemic.[13]

This event had at least one fortunate outcome in that it accelerated the introduction of vaccination programs in many countries, including the United States. In New York City, the Health Department appointed an inspector of vaccinations, supported by a twelve-person staff, and performed 126,003 smallpox vaccinations in 1874 alone.[14] There were nonetheless 1,280 deaths from smallpox in the city during the following year, when the epidemic peaked. In subsequent years, the number of deaths from the disease was much lower, despite the fact that the Health Department was unable to compel vaccination and still had to confront a formidable antivaccination movement.[15]

---

12 Paul Saunders, *Edward Jenner: The Cheltenham Years, 1795–1823* (Hanover, NH, 1982), pp. 7–63.

13 Chase, *Magic Shots*, pp. 47–75. Genevieve Miller, *The Adoption of Inoculation for Smallpox in England and France* (Philadelphia, 1957).

14 The Health Department replaced the Metropolitan Board of Health in 1870. Duffy, *Public Health in New York City*, p. 51. See ibid., p. 71 on the smallpox vaccination program. In addition to the vaccinations, the Department distributed vaccination quill points (13,826) to charitable organizations and sold more than $1,200 worth of the virus.

15 Ibid., pp. 148–54. The state did require that all children admitted to school be vaccinated, but this regulation was frequently ignored. J. Duffy, "School Vaccination: The Precursor to School Medical Inspection," *Journal of the History of Medicine and Allied Sciences* 33 (1978): 344–55. There were instances of enforced vaccination of adults, but that appears to have been the exception, not the rule, as

3

Insofar as the resistance to vaccination was a product of a lack of understanding, the research of Pasteur, Koch, and their cohorts of scientists – including Elie Metchnikoff (1845–1916), Paul Ehrlich (1854–1915), and Emil von Behring (1854–1917) – provided a solid rationale for this means of preventing disease. Metchnikoff uncovered the basic nature of phagocytosis and, in Frankfurt, Ehrlich developed the theoretical basis for the chemical nature of immunity and chemotherapy.[16] As yet, the viral etiology of smallpox had not been discovered. But where bacterial disease was concerned, a rush of discoveries in the 1880s and 1890s laid the foundation for the rapid expansion of vaccinology, for the growth of the public health movement, and for the entrepreneurial efforts of pioneering biological firms like the H. K. Mulford Company.

The attention of both Mulford's executives and New York's new Division of Pathology, Bacteriology, and Disinfection was aroused

---

late as the 1890s. See C. E. Rosenberg, "Making It in Urban Medicine: A Career in the Age of Scientific Medicine," *Bulletin of the History of Medicine* 64, no. 2 (1990): 177. The Department began in the 1870s and 1880s to produce its own pure vaccine. It took this step in part because of concerns about contamination of the vaccine matter and in part because of an inability to obtain sufficient supplies during the epidemic.

16 On Metchnikoff, see Alfred I. Tauber and Leon Chernyak, *Metchnikoff and the Origins of Immunology* (New York, 1991), pp. 101–74; Elie Metchnikoff, *Immunity in Infectious Diseases* (New York, 1968 [1905]). On Ehrlich, see Ernst Bäumler, *Paul Ehrlich: Scientist for Life* (New York, 1984), pp. 47–67; also see Paul Ehrlich, *Collected Papers of Paul Ehrlich*, 3 vols. (London, 1956–60). On Behring, see Wesley W. Spink, *Infectious Diseases: Prevention and Treatment in the Nineteenth and Twentieth Centuries* (Minneapolis, 1978), pp. 170–1.

On all three and the immunological contexts in which their work developed, see Silverstein, *History of Immunology*, pp. 38-123; Pauline Mazumdar, ed., *Immunology, 1930–1980: Essays on the History of Immunology* (Toronto, 1989); P. Mazumdar, "Immunity in 1890," *Journal of the History of Medicine and Allied Sciences* 27 (1972): 312–24. As Silverstein explains, phagocytosis is the ingestion by a cell of another cell or particle (p. 390).

when the news reached America in the early 1890s of a promising new treatment for diphtheria.[17] Emil von Behring and Shibasaburo Kitasato (1852–1931), a Japanese postdoctoral researcher, had analyzed the toxin-destroying ability of blood serum taken from immunized animals and coined the word "antitoxin."[18] In 1891, von Behring and another colleague presented a paper in London that explained how blood serum from artificially immunized animals could be used to combat the exotoxins[19] of the diphtheria bacilli. Three years later, Emile Roux of the Pasteur Institute presented an address to the Eighth International Congress of Hygiene and Demography (Budapest) that made "the healing power of diphtheria antitoxin . . . the foremost medical question of the day."[20] By that time, a German firm in Höchst was already producing a promising diphtheria antitoxin.[21] Both the New York Health Department and the Philadelphia pharmaceutical company were alert to these important signals coming from abroad.

---

17 J. McFarland, "The Beginning of Bacteriology in Philadelphia: Recollections of What Took Place Before the Beginning of the Present Century, with Contemporary Portraits and a Bibliography of the Literature of That Period," *Bulletin of the Institute of the History of Medicine* 5, no. 2 (1937): 184.

18 E. von Behring and S. Kitasato, "Über das Zustandekommen der Diphtherie-Immunität und der Tetanus-Immunität bei Thieren," *Deutsche Medicinische Wochenschrift* 16, no. 49 (1890): 1113-14; E. von Behring, "Untersuchungen über das Zustandekommen der Diphtherie-Immunität bei Thieren," *Deutsche Medicinische Wochenschrift* 16, no. 50 (1890): 1145–8. R. R. MacGregor, "Corynebacterium Diphtheriae," in Gerald L. Mandell, R. Gordon Douglas, Jr., and John E. Bennett, eds., *Principles and Practice of Infectious Diseases*, 3rd ed. (New York, 1990), pp. 1574–81; Henry James Parish, *Victory with Vaccines: The Story of Immunization* (Edinburgh, 1968), pp. 44–51; Chase, *Magic Shots*, pp. 154–77.

19 The word *exotoxin* was originally used to refer to all toxins produced and released by gram-positive bacteria during growth.

20 M. E. Roux, "Sur les serums antitoxiques," *Annales de l'Institut Pasteur* 8 (1894): 722–7. The quotation is from W. H. Welch, "The Treatment of Diphtheria by Antitoxin," *Bulletin of the Johns Hopkins Hospital* 6, nos. 52–3 (1895): 98.

21 Wade W. Oliver, *The Man Who Lived for Tomorrow: A Biography of William Hallock Park, M.D.* (New York, 1941), pp. 45–6.

CHAPTER 2

THE MULFORD STORY

P HILADELPHIA had a well-established pharmaceutical industry in the nineteenth century, but it was not at all clear that one of the city's firms would become the early commercial leader in the biological network that was beginning to develop in the United States. Nor was the H. K. Mulford Company the obvious choice to be the first firm to bring a new serum treatment for diphtheria to market. Other firms in Philadelphia had been in the business longer, were larger, had greater resources, and should no doubt have led the way in developing this new capability.[1] New York City – the other leading medical center in the United States – also had a number of pharmaceutical producers. They had

---

1 On the development of firm capabilities – a major theme throughout this book – see Alfred D. Chandler, Jr., *Scale and Scope: The Dynamics of Industrial Capitalism* (Cambridge, MA, 1990), especially pp. 14–46; while Chandler's emphasis is upon very large corporations, there is in his work an implicit comparison between large and small organizations. In the case at hand, the H. K. Mulford Company, economies of scale and scope favored other firms in the industry. See also the following: D. Teece and G. Pisano, "The Dynamic Capabilities of Firms: An Introduction," *Industrial and Corporate Change* 3, no. 3 (1994): 537–56; the entire issue of the journal is devoted to "dynamic capabilities." G. Dosi and L. Marengo, "Some Elements of an Evolutionary Theory of Organizational Competences," in R. W. England, ed., *Evolutionary Concepts in Contemporary Economics* (Ann Arbor, 1994), pp. 157–78. R. R. Nelson, "Why Do Firms Differ, and How Does It Matter?" *Strategic Management Journal* 12, special issue (1991): 61–74.

the advantage of proximity to the Board of Health's Division of Pathology, Bacteriology, and Disinfection, one of the formative organizations in this particular network.

1

In this instance, however, neither abundant resources nor location appeared to convey any significant commercial advantages, but the entrepreneurial instincts of Mulford's president and vice president did.[2] The vice president, Henry K. Mulford, had established the firm in the late 1880s, when he purchased the "Old Simes" drugstore at the corner of 18th and Market Streets in downtown Philadelphia. The drugstore, which dated back to 1815, had been operated by two well established pharmacists, Joseph L. Remington and Lucius P. Sayre. Remington was dean of the Philadelphia College of Pharmacy and had published a text, *Remington's Practice of Pharmacy*, that went through sixteen editions after its initial appearance in 1885. After selling the store to Mulford, his former employee, Sayre became dean of the College of Pharmacy at the University of Kansas.[3]

Although Mulford was only twenty-one when he took over, he was not content running a retail drugstore. Shortly after he acquired the business, he began to produce a line of pharmaceutical preparations, including lozenges, elixirs, tinctures, antiseptics, fluid extracts, and liquors, along with syrups for the burgeoning soda

---

2 Because the development of the new therapy was so recent and so poorly understood, it seems likely that the risk of moving into biologicals at this early date discouraged some of the larger, better established companies. Neither the depression following 1893 nor the risks involved, however, discouraged Parke-Davis & Company of Detroit, which was also quick to move into the new field.

While location favored New York over Philadelphia, both urban centers had important medical resources and personnel; in that sense, location *was* a factor. The innovation did not take place in rural New Hampshire, for obvious reasons.

3 See the obituary for H. K. Mulford in the *North Western Druggist* (Dec. 1937): 59–60. In addition to working for Sayre and Remington, Mulford trained at the Philadelphia College of Pharmacy.

fountain trade. This was the traditional route followed by pharmaceutical entrepreneurs, and by the 1880s, there were more than 140 such firms in Philadelphia, most of them selling both to the wholesale and retail drug trade, as Mulford was.[4]

Short of working capital and determined to expand his operations, Mulford sought a financial backer and found it in 1889 in the person of Milton Campbell, a fellow graduate of the Philadelphia College of Pharmacy.[5] The two men needed only a thirty-minute conversation to cement their relationship. In 1891 they reorganized and incorporated the H. K. Mulford Company, with Campbell as president and Mulford as vice president.[6] The firm had net assets of about $46,000 at that time.[7] During the following year, they had sales of only $35,000, but they broadened their product line and made good use of a compressed tablet machine that Mulford and a colleague patented. Their mass-produced, water-soluble pills found a ready market, and soon the H. K. Mulford Company was operating two laboratories for the production of a greatly expanded line of "pills and medicinal agents." By this time, they were marketing more than 800 different medical products[8] and had a branch office in Chicago.[9]

---

4 Fehr Ms., pp. 1–2, in Merck Archives, hereafter MA; Liebenau, *Medical Science and Medical Industry*, pp. 11–24, 57–8.

5 *The Keystone*, Dec. 20, 1918, MA. This publication was for a time the Mulford Company's newsletter.

6 Fehr Ms., p. 2; Beard editorial, "All About Us," c. 1928, pp. 1–2; both in MA.

7 "Mulford Co. Minutes – 1891 to 1896," MA.

8 H. K. Mulford Company, "Prospectus," n.d.; H. K. Mulford Co., Price-List, Oct. 1893; both in MA. We classified as different products the various combinations of drugs – for example, Aconite versus Aconite and Belladonna – sold by the company.

9 Liebenau, *Medical Science and Medical Industry*, pp. 57-8. *Bulletin of the Philadelphia College of Pharmacy*, Aug. 1947; and H. K. Mulford Co., Price-List, Book #2, n.d.; both in MA.

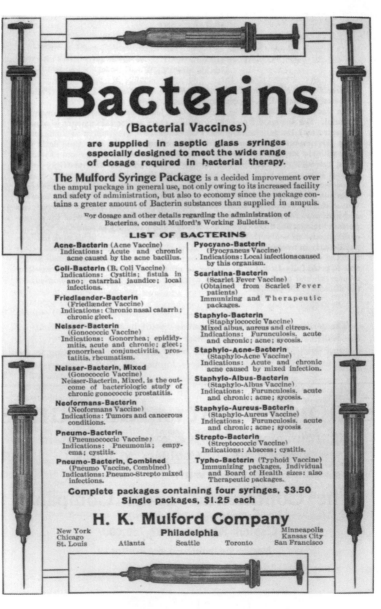

In 1894, Campbell and Mulford decided to attempt a far more dramatic innovation than the tablet machine. They had noted with interest the publicity about a new diphtheria antitoxin. The University of Pennsylvania had recently established a new hygiene laboratory, where the staff taught and researched the recent developments in bacteriology, as did their counterparts at the Medico-Chirurgical College in Philadelphia and the new Pepper Clinical Laboratory of the University Hospital. Although the Municipal Health Department had lagged behind New York in this new field, the news about diphtheria antitoxin stimulated a "public clamor" for similar efforts in Philadelphia.[10] The department responded by organizing a new hygiene laboratory.[11]

Neither Campbell nor Mulford was trained in the new medical science, but they recognized the opportunities embodied in the "clamor" for diphtheria antitoxin and moved decisively to position the H. K. Mulford Company to become a leader in the new field. Realizing that they needed scientific expertise, they met in the late autumn of 1894 with Dr. Joseph McFarland, who was a lecturer on bacteriology and pathological histology in the University of Pennsylvania's Medical Department. McFarland, who was also teaching part-time at the Philadelphia Polyclinic and College for Graduates in Medicine, had studied

---

10 See E. M. Hammonds, "Wars Against Disease: Anti-Diphtheria Campaigns and the Media" (paper presented at The Seminar, Department of History, The Johns Hopkins University, Mar. 7, 1994). See also Terra Ziporyn, *Disease in the Popular American Press: The Case of Diphtheria, Typhoid Fever, and Syphilis, 1870–1920* (New York, 1988), pp. 41–53.

11 J. McFarland, "The Beginning of Bacteriology in Philadelphia: Recollections of What Took Place Before the Beginning of the Present Century, with Contemporary Portraits and a Bibliography of the Literature of That Period," *Bulletin of the Institute of the History of Medicine* 5, no. 2 (1937): 158–70, 172–4, 177–83. The most authoritative source is E. T. Morman, "Scientific Medicine Comes to Philadelphia: Public Health Transformed, 1854–1899" (Ph.D. diss., University of Pennsylvania, 1986), especially pp. 148–240. Morman's account differs in several regards from the narrative in Liebenau, *Medical Science and Medical Industry*.

bacteriology in Heidelberg and Vienna. He had been following the scientific literature from Europe and was also familiar with what had been accomplished in the laboratory of the New York City Board of Health. Campbell and Mulford promptly offered him a position with their firm, assuring him that he could do this job in his "spare time." McFarland, who had been supporting himself with part-time teaching jobs, quickly accepted at a salary of $100 a month. It took the Board of Directors of the corporation only three days to decide to support this new venture, even though money was so tight they would need to sell 100 shares of stock in order to finance the operation.[12]

While the company was eager to provide McFarland with a small staff and a "Biological Laboratory," what their new director of research most needed was detailed information about the process of producing effective serum antitoxin. McFarland's initial staff included Clarence W. Lincoln (also in pathological histology) and John Adams (professor of surgery in the University of Pennsylvania's Veterinary Department), neither of whom "had ever performed any of the tasks confronting" them. They knew from the scientific literature that horses had been inoculated with gradually increasing doses of diphtheria toxin, isolated from cultures of the bacillus grown in vitro. When the horses became "hyperimmune," their blood contained massive quantities of antibodies to diphtheria. The horses were then carefully bled through the jugular vein, and the serum was separated from the clot by straining.[13] But

---

12 Morman, "Scientific Medicine," p. 184. "Mulford Co. Minutes – 1891 to 1896," MA. Liebenau, *Medical Science and Medical Industry*, pp. 58–9, gives a slightly different account of McFarland's background. The firm's shortage of capital and the failure of its larger rivals to move quickly into biological production may both have been related to the nationwide economic depression that had begun in 1893.

13 For a review of the early literature available to McFarland see W. H. Welch, "The Treatment of Diphtheria by Antitoxin," *Bulletin of the Johns Hopkins Hospital* 6, nos. 52–3 (1895): 97–8. The horses could not contract diphtheria, and the company employed the veterinarian John Adams to ensure that the bleeding was done without injury to the animals.

McFarland still needed to know exactly "what to do and how to do it." And he needed virulent diphtheria toxin in large quantities.[14]

For help he turned to William Park, M.D., Bacteriological Diagnostician of Diphtheria for the New York City Health Department. Park (like McFarland) had studied in Europe and upon returning to the United States had concentrated his research efforts on diphtheria. By 1894, he had helped create New York's system of depots at which physicians could obtain kits for diagnosing and recording diphtheria cases.[15] That same year, his boss, Dr. Herman M. Biggs, visited the Koch Institute in Germany and learned firsthand how diphtheria antitoxin was being prepared. Park was at work from that point on, producing serum antitoxin for use in New York and encouraging others to adopt this new treatment.[16] Very soon, Park and his colleagues were making important practical contributions to the therapy by developing stronger serums than were being used in Europe. The advantage of having multiple centers of experimentation and development was apparent in this network as early as the 1890s.[17]

When approached by McFarland, Park was heavily engaged in developing the facilities for producing antitoxin, but he nevertheless took the time to provide Mulford's researcher with the detailed informa-

---

14 McFarland, "Beginning of Bacteriology," p. 186.

15 Oliver, *Man Who Lived For Tomorrow*, pp. 24–8, 52–63, 75–97.

16 Ibid., pp. 98–125. Duffy, *Public Health in New York City*, pp. 99–101. Both sources discuss the *New York Herald* campaign to raise money to support this effort. See also M. Schaeffer, "William H. Park (1863–1939): His Laboratory and His Legacy," *American Journal of Public Health* 75, no. 11 (1985): 1296–1302.

17 Although he deals with a much later period in the development of the industry, Alfonso Gambardella comes to a similar conclusion in *Science and Innovation*, pp. 166–7. An excellent example of the contrary situation, one in which only one center existed, is provided by the saga of poor Oliver Heaviside and his attempts to convince the British General Post Office to adopt his theory of transmission. Neil H. Wasserman, *From Invention to Innovation: Long-Distance Telephone Transmission at the Turn of the Century* (Baltimore, 1985), pp. 21–30.

tion and the cultures needed to get the operation started.[18] Although McFarland was representing a commercial organization, the two men had similar educational backgrounds and shared a common orientation toward scientific progress in medicine. Personal relationships and this kind of cooperative behavior were important elements in the complex process of innovation taking place in the 1890s. In later years, when institutional settings became more bureaucratic and relationships more formal, communication would no longer be as simple as it was when McFarland visited Dr. Park's laboratory.

On his return to Philadelphia, McFarland and his associates tried to put into practice the lessons they had learned. It took time to develop an appropriate culture medium, to acquire the right kind of equipment, and to discover how to keep the cultures from becoming contaminated. "The importance of expedition [had] . . . been emphasized," he later commented, "but almost everything that we did seemed destined to retard our progress." Their laboratory was on the second floor of a large stable in West Philadelphia, and the atmosphere of the stable was not conducive to bacteriological work. While McFarland struggled through the winter of 1894–5, William Park had made the first use (January 1, 1895) of his lab's antitoxin to treat two cases of diphtheria in New York.[19] By the late spring, others were at work as well, including Parke-Davis, the large Detroit pharmaceutical firm.[20]

For McFarland and his colleagues these were tense months of experimentation. When at last they were able to obtain a reasonable output of serum antitoxin, they still needed help. Lacking the facilities to test the antitoxin, McFarland turned to the Laboratory of Hygiene at

18 McFarland, "Beginning of Bacteriology," p. 186. McFarland had also talked to Dr. Gibier of the Pasteur Institute in New York.

19 Duffy, *Public Health in New York City*, p. 100. Oliver, *Man Who Lived For Tomorrow*, p. 109.

20 Liebenau, *Medical Science and Medical Industry*, pp. 59–60. "The Beginning of Laboratory Research," in *Parke-Davis At 100* (Detroit, 1966).

*A Mulford delivery
truck, c. 1915.*

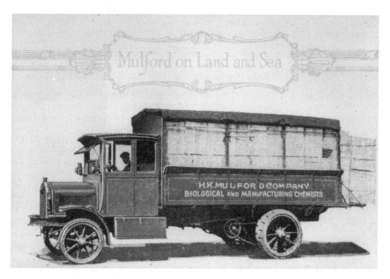

the University of Pennsylvania for assistance. The University laboratory
tested his product and in the early summer of 1895, H. K. Mulford was
able to offer for sale the first commercial diphtheria antitoxin produced
in the United States.[21] That accomplishment was a credit to an entrepreneurial firm but also to the innovative network of public and private
organizations in which Mulford was now strategically positioned.

21 For the next two years, the University tested every lot of Mulford antitoxin.
This type of loosely organized university/industry cooperation would become very
common in the United States during the twentieth century. It would become a
central feature of Merck's operations in the years following 1930, when the firm
established its first modern research and development organization. John P.
Swann, *Academic Scientists and the Pharmaceutical Industry: Cooperative Research in
Twentieth-Century America* (Baltimore, 1988), especially pp. 24–39. See also Chapter 5.

The links between the universities and the companies appear to have
been partly professional in nature and partly financial. For tiny companies like
Mulford, the cost of additional personnel and equipment seems to have precluded
bringing this function within the firm at this time.

The firm continued to look to this system of institutions for the resources and ideas it needed to push forward in biologicals. Mulford
hired Professor Leonard Pearson, who had studied with Koch in Germany, from the Veterinary School at the University of Pennsylvania.
Staff members with good professional credentials strengthened the company's claim that it was a scientifically advanced organization. Though
the techniques for producing antitoxin – it was, for instance, strained
through cheese cloth – seem to us unbelievably crude, Mulford's laboratory was by the standards of that day an unusually meticulous commercial organization. As the price-list noted, "Everything has been
conducted on a strictly careful and scientific basis, and we take just
pride in being one of the first to produce a reliable Serum in America.
The standardizing of our products is not only carefully carried out in
our own laboratory, but is also confirmed by the Department of Hygiene, of the University of Pennsylvania, each package being dated and
stamped with its strength expressed in immunity units." To reinforce
this claim, the firm opened its laboratories and stables to the inspection
of the medical profession one day a month.[22]

The inspections, the quality of the staff, and the commitment
of the partners to scientific standards convinced others that Mulford's
claims were more substantial than the usual advertising statements.
These claims were further strengthened after 1896, when the company's executives moved the biological operations to Glenolden, Pennsylvania, eight miles outside Philadelphia. There the company built
laboratories for biological, veterinary, and vaccine work, as well as a
large stable and cow barn. Now McFarland's biological lab was separated from the stables and the contamination they inevitably introduced. After the facility was inspected by the Pennsylvania State Board
of Health, the company noted that "the report gives an exceedingly
high standing to the biological laboratory and stables of the H. K.
Mulford Company, of Philadelphia, the stables being scrupulously

22 H. K. Mulford Company, Price-List, Oct. 1, 1895, MA.

clean, the animals sound and vigorous, the laboratory arrangements good, the technique careful and thorough, and the product of somewhat greater strength than advertised. This assertion could not be made of all the European products."[23]

Standardization was a major issue at that time. Behring and Ehrlich were developing adequate techniques for standardizing antitoxin, and Mulford quickly became a leader (with Parke-Davis) in this important technical development. The company's analytical laboratory was well equipped, and the firm's reputation for careful standardization became an important asset.[24]

Technical innovation led the firm to adopt new techniques in marketing and sales, approaches oriented to a specific segment of the market. Through its advertising and educational campaigns, the Mulford Company reached out to the medical profession throughout the United States. Merck & Co., in New York, listed Mulford's antitoxin in *Merck's 1896 Index*, an encyclopedia for pharmacists, doctors, dentists, veterinarians, and chemists.[25] Mulford also developed monographs and other publications, made lantern slides, and produced "moving picture films" for educational institutions, boards of education, and the medical

---

23 *Twelfth Annual Report of Secretary of Pennsylvania State Board of Health, Nov. 12, 1986*, as quoted in H. K. Mulford Company, Price-List, Sept. 1897, MA. See also Liebenau, *Medical Science and Medical Industry*, p. 63; the author notes that the price-list for 1900 quotes the *Philadelphia Medical Times*: "Manufacturers of this character deserve unstinted commendation as public benefactors. The laboratories of the H. K. Mulford Company are, in point of scientific equipment, the most complete in existence, and are under the immediate personal control of eminent scientists." Even after applying a normal discount for journalistic exaggeration ("most complete" and "eminent"), one can conclude that the operation had acquired an excellent reputation in circles that mattered to the firm.

24 See, for instance, H. K. Mulford Company, Price-List, 1897, MA.

25 There was a full-page advertisement for the Mulford antitoxin in the 1896 *Index* (p. 120a); Merck also listed the imported antitoxins by Aronson, Behring, Pasteur, and Roux (p. 42). Merck had apparently been supplying the American trade with the Behring product since early 1895. *Merck's Market Report*, Jan. 15, 1895, MA.

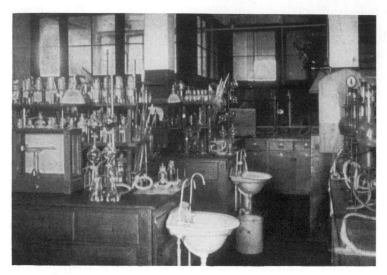

and pharmaceutical colleges. These media advertised the firm while they informed the profession and the public about the dangers of diphtheria and the most advanced methods for treating the disease.

As the advertising material explained, Mulford's serum provided what Paul Ehrlich labeled "passive" (short-term) immunity. In the case of "active" immunity, as with smallpox vaccination, antigens stimulated the body to produce antibodies and provide long-lasting or permanent immunity. Mulford's antiserum product worked by temporarily neutralizing or counteracting the effects of the diphtheria toxins.[26] Given the fact that as late as 1890–3, one-third to one-half of the hospitalized diphtheria patients died from the disease, it was a great advance to be able, using serum antitoxin, to cut the death rate in half.[27]

26 Mulford Guide Book, p. 16. MA.

27 Anne Hardy, *The Epidemic Streets: Infectious Disease and the Rise of Preventive Medicine, 1856–1900* (Oxford, 1993), pp. 95–6. Oliver, *Man Who Lived For Tomorrow*, pp. 116–17. Welch, "Treatment of Diphtheria," especially pp. 103–

As might be imagined, Mulford's success with its first antitoxin encouraged the company to stay in touch with the fast-moving frontiers of immunology and to experiment with other biologicals for treating or preventing disease. McFarland's second success was with tetanus antitoxin, which the company sold in both human and veterinary dosages.[28] In 1898, Mulford added Dr. W. F. Elgin to the laboratory staff and gave him the responsibility for moving the firm into the development of a smallpox vaccine; by August of that year, Mulford was selling "glycerinated vaccine lymph" and the scarifiers used to administer the vaccine.[29]

By 1904, when the federal government granted Mulford li-

---

12. American practice on dosages was more aggressive than that of European physicians, and this apparently accounts to some degree for the quick success of the new therapy in the United States; see A. Hardy, "Tracheotomy Versus Intubation: Surgical Intervention in Diphtheria in Europe and the United States, 1825–1930," *Bulletin of the History of Medicine* 66, no. 4 (1992): 554–5.

28 H. K. Mulford Company, Price-List, Apr. 1897, MA. By this time, McFarland's laboratory was able to produce culture media (Loeffler's blood serum mixture) for use in bacteriological work, and the company was also selling an improved antitoxin syringe. See also McFarland, "Beginning of Bacteriology," p. 188.

In 1899, Mulford brought out two new veterinary products: an anthrax vaccine and a vaccine for black-leg disease. H. K. Mulford Company, Price-List, Oct. 1899. The company later produced a serum treatment for anthrax that was also used in the rare cases in which humans contracted the disease. A. D. Melvin to the Surgeon General, Oct. 8 and 19, 1915; A. Eichhorn to Surgeon General Rupert Blue, Oct. 19, 1915, with enclosure; A. Eichhorn, "Vaccination Experiments Against Anthrax," c. 1915; all in Record Group 90, at the U.S. National Archives (hereafter RG 90, NA).

29 H. K. Mulford Company, Price-List, Aug. 1898, MA. Dr. W. F. Elgin, "A Quarter Century of Vaccine Production with H. K. Mulford Co.," manuscript, MA. As Elgin pointed out, the firm also introduced process innovations, learning for instance how to keep the glycerinated virus in cold storage. He estimated that the firm sold about 45 million of the vaccination tube points between 1898 and 1914.

cense No. 2 to manufacture antitoxins and vaccines (under the 1902 Biologicals Control Act[30]), the firm was selling serum for anthrax, dysentery, melitensis (also called undulant or Malta fever; today, brucellosis[31]), meningitis, pneumonia, streptococcal infections, and tetanus, as well as the original diphtheria serum.[32] Though there was no reliable clinical evidence for the efficacy of some of the serums, there were few alternative treatments. Given the seriousness of these illnesses, one can understand why the serums were widely employed.[33]

Mulford had also become a leading producer of vaccines.[34] It was doing a substantial business in smallpox vaccine, using calf lymph; and by 1911 it was producing rabies vaccine, using the Pasteur method.[35] It was also making the so-called bacterins and serobacterins

---

30 J. F. Anderson to the Surgeon General, Sept. 12, 1904; and H. D. Geddings, et al., to the Surgeon General, Nov. 1, 1907; in RG 90, NA. See also R. A. Kondratas, "Biologics Control Act of 1902," in James Harvey Young, ed., *The Early Years of Federal Food and Drug Control* (Madison, WI, 1982), pp. 8–27. Mulford's major competitor, Parke-Davis & Co., received license No. 1.

31 See D. J. Mikolich and J. M. Boyce, "Brucella Species," in Mandell, Douglas, and Bennett, eds., *Infectious Diseases*, pp. 1735–42.

32 See the report of the Surgeon Inspector to the Surgeon General on Mulford's vaccine production [1904]; and J. F. Anderson to the Surgeon General, Oct. 30, 1905, reporting on an inspection of Mulford's facilities; on anthrax serum see J. F. Anderson to the Surgeon General, July 8, 1913; all in RG 90, NA.

33 The company also sold various biological products for use in laboratory and clinical tests. These included various forms of culture media, agglutinating serum for diagnosis of cholera, and diphtheria toxin for the Schick test. H. K. Mulford Company, Price-List, May 1904, MA.

34 Vaccination is a prophylactic immunization. It involves the "induction of long-term . . . immunity against infectious diseases by the injection or oral ingestion of whole live, altered, or inactivated microbial pathogens; or antigens removed from the structures of microbes; or toxoids made by chemically altering bacterial toxins." Chase, *Magic Shots*, p. 559.

35 The rabies vaccine used the attenuated virus prepared from the spinal cord of an animal infected with rabies. H. K. Mulford Company, "Biological Products," pp. 46–8, MA. The company supplied a "Mulford Rabies Vaccine Outfit" that

---

("sensitized bacterial vaccines" in the advertising). Bacterins consisted of killed bacteria (that is, antigens) and were designed to produce active immunity by stimulating the formation of specific antibodies following parenteral injection.[36] The serobacterins combined killed bacteria (antigens) and the antibodies of an immune serum. They were an attempt to combine the short-term action of the serums with the (presumably) lasting action of the bacterins. The H. K. Mulford Company experimented with a large number of bacterins and serobacterins, ranging from those used for acne and hay fever to those employed for treating cholera, staphylococcal infections, and typhoid fever.[37] Along the way, the company also developed a new aseptic piston syringe package; and an aseptic, sealed glass container/scarifier for administering smallpox vaccinations.[38]

During the years that followed, Mulford and the medical profession gradually began to sort out the effective from some of the ineffective antitoxin and vaccine treatments. This was a slow and difficult process, in large part because of the state of knowledge of immunology at the time. There was, for example, a theoretical basis for the use of bacterins. They were thought to produce an increase in the

contained all of the equipment needed for a full series of treatments. A. P. Hitchens to Dr. John F. Anderson, Mar. 16, 1911; L. E. Cofer, et al., to the Surgeon General, Apr. 13 and 29, 1911; W. Wyman to H. K. Mulford Company, May 8, 1911; all in RG 90, NA.

36 Parenteral injections are all of those that put substances into the body other than through the digestive canal.

37 For a product such as antityphoid vaccine, Mulford had six competitors in the United States in 1912. They were Parke-Davis & Co.; the National Vaccine and Antitoxin Institute (Washington, D.C.); Lederle Antitoxin Laboratories; The Cutter Laboratory; Burroughs, Wellcome & Co.; and the Swiss Serum and Vaccine Institute, whose American agents were the Pasteur Laboratories of America. J. W. Kerr to Dr. R. C. Lamson, Sept. 10, 1912, RG 90, NA.

38 H. K. Mulford Company, "Biological Products," especially pp. 31, 42–5, 49–51; "Serobacterins," Bulletin No. 18; Treasury Department to H. K. Mulford Company, Mar. 27, 1916, with enclosed copy of the Mulford license, all in MA.

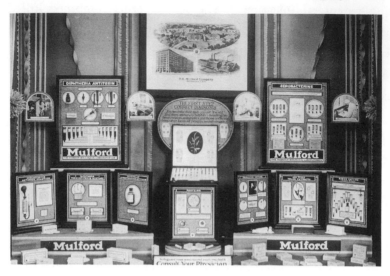

"opsonins," serum substances that prepared invading bacteria for phagocytosis. The clinical evidence in support of this theory was mixed, but it was not until the late 1930s and early 1940s that the therapy went into decline.[39]

5

Meanwhile, companies like Mulford had experienced substantial growth and developed significant new capabilities as producers and

---

39 The theory of opsonins is still correct for encapsulated bacteria such as pneumococci. But see P. Keating, "Vaccine Therapy and the Problem of Opsonins," *Journal of the History of Medicine and Allied Sciences*, 43 (1988): 275–96. Other new serum products included an antiplague serobacterin, for which the company was planning a new building in 1915. See A. P. Atchens to the Surgeon General, July 23, 1915, with enclosures; the Surgeon General to H. K. Mulford Company, Aug. 9, 1915, RG 90, NA. The Surgeon Inspector's report to the Surgeon General (1912) on Mulford's streptococcal bacterin said: "The use of these sensitized 'bacterial vaccines' prepared after the method of Besredka rests on good experimental basis." In RG 90, NA.

distributors of these and other biologicals. The firm grew to an impressive size: by 1902, annual sales were more than $1 million; by 1910, it had 950 employees and was grossing about $3 million a year.[40] By this time, Joseph McFarland had left the company to return to teaching and research; his position had been filled temporarily by Clarence W. Lincoln and then by Dr. Joseph James Kinyoun, who had formerly headed the Washington laboratory of the U.S. Public Health Service.[41] In 1911, Dr. Oswald Avery would help introduce the staff to the latest techniques in bacteriology, and later, Dr. John Reichel, who had received his training at the University of Pennsylvania, would become head of research.[42]

---

40 The distribution capabilities of the private organizations were important. To the Midwest and South, in the more agrarian parts of the country, public health facilities on balance lagged behind those of the large urban centers of the East Coast. See, for example, the experience of Minnesota with smallpox and diphtheria: Philip D. Jordan, *The People's Health: A History of Public Health in Minnesota to 1948* (Saint Paul, 1953), pp. 398–409. See also J. Duffy, "School Vaccination: The Precursor to School Medical Inspection," *Journal of the History of Medicine and Allied Sciences* 33 (1978): 344–55. Charles V. Chapin, *A Report on State Public Health Work Based on a Survey of State Boards of Health* (Chicago, [1915]), table 1.

41 Harden, *Inventing the NIH*, pp. 13–15. See also Edward Shorter, *The Health Century* (New York, 1987), pp. 6–7. Kinyoun had established the original laboratory on Staten Island at the Marine Hospital. Williams, *U.S. Public Health Service*, pp. 176–81. In 1907, Kinyoun left Mulford to become professor of pathology and bacteriology at the George Washington University Medical School. Williams, *U.S. Public Health Service*, p. 249.

42 Avery would later move to the Rockefeller Institute and would be a codiscoverer of the chemical basis of heredity. Avery, et al., would identify and define the "transforming chemical – it was 'a nucleic acid of the deoxyribose (DNA) type.' " Chase, *Magic Shots*, pp. 223, 234. Liebenau, *Medical Science and Medical Industry*, pp. 67, 73; H. K. Mulford Company, "Prospectus, with the History, Growth and Development of the H. K. Mulford Company, Incorporated"; "Drug and Cosmetic Industry," May 1938, p. 623; W. F. Elgin, "A Quarter Century of Vaccine Production with H. K. Mulford Co."; all in MA. For a time, Dr. W. F. Elgin, who had (with one brief interruption) directed the smallpox vaccine operation since 1898, would be in charge of the entire laboratory.

Under their leadership, Mulford's laboratories made substantial progress in improving the firm's products, for example, by developing new techniques to increase the potency of the popular diphtheria antitoxin and to lengthen its shelf life. Centrifuges and "germ-free filters" replaced the cheesecloth strainers, and the well-equipped, well-staffed Mulford laboratories were generally acknowledged to be at least the equal of any in the industry.[43] The company's reputation was a significant asset, and when production problems arose — as they did in 1909 — Mulford was quick to correct the situation. At both Parke-Davis and Mulford, hoof and mouth disease in their vaccine herds contaminated the companies' vaccines in 1909. After removing the products from the market, destroying the infected animals, and eliminating the contamination, Mulford and its chief competitor were authorized to restore production.[44]

The quality of its products and the firm's strong scientific reputation paid off during World War I. Even before the United States

---

43 The best guides to the technical changes taking place are the U.S. Public Health Service reports based on regular inspections; these reports describe in detail the production processes from 1904 on; these are in RG 90, NA. See also H. K. Mulford Company, *Antitoxins and Vaccine*, c. 1901; *Mulford's Diphtheria Antitoxin*, c. 1903; both in Library, College of Physicians of Philadelphia, hereafter LCPP. Later, Mulford developed a combined toxin-antitoxin or "toxoid," which became the standard vaccine for diphtheria. Chase, *Magic Shots*, p. 200.

44 Surgeon M. J. Rosenau to the Surgeon General, Mar. 12 and May 17, 1909; H. D. Geddings, et al., to the Surgeon General, Mar. 16, 1909; H. K. Mulford to Dr. M. J. Rosenau, Apr. 8, 1909; J. F. Anderson to the Surgeon General, Apr. 12 and 13, and Nov. 11, 1909; J. B. Reynolds to H. K. Mulford Company, Apr. 15, 1909; W. Wyman to the Secretary of the Treasury, Aug. 12, 1909; C. D. Norton to Surgeon M. J. Rosenau, Aug. 23, 1909; all in RG 90, NA. Another problem arose in December of 1910 and was also quickly corrected. See Assistant Secretary to John F. Anderson, Dec. 20, 1910; to H. K. Mulford Company, Dec. 21, 1910; J. F. Anderson to the Surgeon General, Dec. 29 and 31, 1909; all in RG 90, NA. See also Liebenau, *Medical Science and Medical Industry*, p. 90.

entered the struggle, Mulford's business quickly tripled.[45] After the U.S. declaration of war in 1917, the government purchased substantial amounts of Mulford diphtheria antitoxin for use by the U.S. Army, and by 1918 the Company had 1,500 horses and 1,200 employees involved in this effort alone.[46] Near the end of that year the firm bought a large building at the corner of Broad and Wallace in Philadelphia to house its enlarged pharmaceutical and business operations, while keeping the biologicals on the spacious site at Glenolden. There were by this time forty-two buildings on Glenolden's 200-acre grounds.[47]

During the prosperous 1920s, Mulford continued to extend its distribution network and to a lesser extent its already extensive product line. By 1925, the company had branch offices in nine major cities in the United States and one in Canada. It had ties with foreign distributors from Africa to Singapore, from Argentina to Spain, New Zealand,

---

45 H. K. Mulford Company to Surgeon General Rupert Blue, Oct. 21, 1914; the Surgeon General to H. K. Mulford Company, Oct. 23, 1914; Royal Italian Government to Dr. Rupert Blue, Sept. 2 and 13, 1916; J. P. Leake to the Surgeon General, Mar. 3 and 14, 1916; B. R. Newton to H. K. Mulford Company, Mar. 27, 1916. In the year 1916–17, Mulford said it had increased capacity by 300 percent; H. K. Mulford Company to Surgeon General Rupert Blue, Apr. 11, 1917. All in RG 90, NA.

46 The company was also supplying other products to the Army; see W. H. Arthur to the Surgeon General, Dec. 21, 1917; M. Kwurzel to the Surgeon General, Jan. 23, 1918, RG 112, NA. Other suppliers of the diphtheria serum included E. R. Squibb & Sons, Lederle Antitoxin Laboratories, Parke-Davis & Co., Slee Laboratories, and United States Standard Serum Co.; see United States Standard Serum Company to Surgeon General, Mar. 27, 1918, and to J. C. O'Mahoney, May 24, 1919; F. X. Strong to United States Standard Serum Company, Mar. 1 and Apr. 16, 1919; Receiving Report No. 192, Jan. 20, 1919; F. X. Strong to H. K. Mulford Company, Feb. 4, 1919; Lederle Antitoxin Laboratories to the Surgeon General, Jan. 25, 1919; F. X. Strong to Parke-Davis & Co., Jan. 31, 1919; Edwin P. Wolfe to the Auditor of the War Department, Feb. 3, 1919; F. X. Strong to Slee Laboratories, Apr. 5, 1919; all in RG 112, NA.

47 *The Keystone*, Dec. 6, 1918 and May 1919, MA; Liebenau, *Medical Science and Medical Industry*, p. 78.

---

and Australia. In that year the company's diphtheria antitoxin was front-page news in the *New York Times*: In January a shipment traveled by dogsled, over 650 miles of ice and snow, from Nenana (at the end of the railroad from Anchorage) to Nome, Alaska, which had been hit by an epidemic of diphtheria.[48] The "race with death" – commemorated today in the Iditarod Trail Dogsled Race – was finished in a raging blizzard; the antitoxin was frozen, but Mulford's president, Milton Campbell, explained to the press that as soon as his firm's product was thawed out it was "ready for use."[49]

In the next few years the company's new product development slowed markedly, but it continued to record substantial sales in biologicals and to penetrate additional markets. By the end of the decade, Mulford was a prime target for the merger movement then sweeping through the chemical and pharmaceutical industries.[50] The company's top executives, Campbell and Mulford, were both in their sixties. Their business had a solid reputation, excellent production capabilities, and a strong set of products. When Sharp & Dohme, a large Baltimore pharmaceutical firm, made a substantial offer to buy the H. K. Mulford Company in 1929, an agreement was quickly arranged.[51]

6

In the years between 1895 and 1929, the Mulford Company had built a substantial business and played an important role in developing and distributing serum antitoxins and vaccines in the United States and abroad. The primary burst of innovative activity in the company and in the private/public network of which it was an important part had taken place in the 1890s. Entrepreneurial activity at Mulford had carried

---

48 *New York Times*, Jan. 30, 1925.

49 *New York Times*, Jan. 29, 30, 31, Feb. 1, 2, 3, 4, 1925.

50 The consolidations of those years included the merger of Merck & Co., Inc., with Powers-Weightman-Rosengarten (another fine-chemical producer) in 1927. For a review of the various consolidations see Williams Haynes, *American Chemical Industry: The Merger Era* (New York, 1948).

51 Ibid., p. 289. H. K. Mulford Company, Price-List, 1929, MA.

An advertisement for
the Mulford syringe.

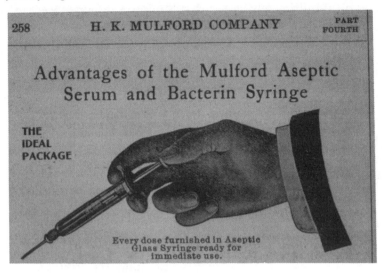

forward into the early 1900s and through World War I, as the firm continued to build capabilities on the foundation provided by the bacteriological revolution in medical science.

Clearly, however, this cycle of innovation was coming to an end some years before the company was sold. Without new and vigorous leadership, without links to emerging areas of medical science, without additional investments in new capabilities, Mulford was fated to remain in a holding pattern — or worse. Like many similar family firms, it could not sustain innovation over the long term.[52] To do so, the Mulford Company would have needed more vigorous executive leadership prepared to guide the organization through a substantial

---

52 There have, of course, been many significant exceptions to this rule. See, for instance, the special issue of *Business History* 35, no. 4 (1993), edited by Geoffrey Jones and Mary B. Rose and dedicated to family capitalism. See also Alfred D. Chandler, Jr., and Stephen Salsbury, *Pierre S. du Pont and the Making of the Modern Corporation* (New York, 1971); and Philip Scranton, *Figured Tapestry: Production, Markets, and Power in Philadelphia Textiles, 1885–1941* (New York, 1989).

scientific and technical transition. Lacking professional management and an appropriate long-term strategy, the firm's owners turned to the market for corporate control, which solved their immediate problems and would ultimately ensure that Mulford's resources were used effectively in a new cycle of innovation.[53]

Despite this ending in 1929, Mulford's single, long cycle of innovation had certainly been a success story. That success was a result of the performance of an entrepreneurial firm and of a complex network of public and private institutions. These institutions were in the 1890s relatively young and undifferentiated. Their boundaries were fluid and their members were, for the most part, more interested in cooperation than competition. Personal and professional ties loomed large. While the participants all had particular motives, they frequently found common ideological ground in the perception that they were exploring a challenging scientific frontier. This was true whether their primary motivation was to make profits, to build scientific careers, or to strengthen the country's public health institutions. By moving quickly and decisively, the H. K. Mulford Company had in 1894 and 1895 become an important part of that dynamic network.

In subsequent decades, both Mulford and the network changed. The public setting acquired a new regulatory function, and from time to time Mulford and its competitors found themselves in conflict with their regulators.[54] On balance, Mulford adapted rela-

---

53 For a treatment of the contemporary market for corporate control see M. C. Jensen, "The Market for Corporate Control," in P. Newman, M. Milgate, and J. Eatwell, eds., *The New Palgrave Dictionary of Money and Finance* (London, 1992), 2:657–66.

54 In addition to the contamination problems noted in the text, there were disagreements over labeling (see, for example, H. K. Mulford to Dr. M. J. Rosenau, Dec. 23, 1907; H. K. Mulford Company to Dr. John F. Anderson, Dec. 28, 1910; W. Wyman to Dr. John Reichel, May 16, 1911; and B. R. Newton to Parke-Davis & Co., et al., Mar. 15, 1915; all in RG 90, NA) and over the efforts to amend the 1902 act providing for federal control of biologicals (see, for example, J. F. Anderson to the Surgeon General, July 8 and Aug. 6, 1914;

tively easily to this new setting, largely because it had from the beginning placed great emphasis on the quality of its research, production, and standardization functions.[55] This was the major way Mulford attempted to differentiate itself from its competitors.[56] The public health organizations were meanwhile becoming more formal and specialized.[57] After a few initial skirmishes, they left the task of producing biologicals largely to the private sector, while concentrating on regulatory functions and on the task of encouraging widespread use of vaccines.[58]

and "Objections to H. R. 13040"; both in RG 90, NA).

55 See Williams, *U.S. Public Health Service*, pp. 182–5. Peter Stechl, "Biological Standardization of Drugs Before 1928" (Ph.D. diss., University of Wisconsin, 1969), especially pp. 47–98, 110–29, 249–50. Liebenau, *Medical Science and Medical Industry*, pp. 90–7.

56 Our conclusion in this regard is based on a careful reading of the company's literature, especially its advertising material, and on the absence of evidence that short-term price competition was particularly important in the firm's markets. The number of competitors was small but there were few opportunities to achieve patent protection. H. K. Mulford's reputation was the primary competitive advantage of this successful firm.

57 M. Waserman, "The Quest for a National Health Department in the Progressive Era," *Bulletin of the History of Medicine* 49, no. 3 (1975): 353–80. Bess Furman, *A Profile of the United States Public Health Service* (Bethesda, MD, 1973), pp. 229–379. Williams, *U.S. Public Health Service*, pp. 118–75, 411–35, 560–611. Harden, *Inventing the NIH*, especially pp. 71–159. Elizabeth Fee, *Disease and Discovery: A History of the Johns Hopkins School of Hygiene and Public Health, 1916–1939* (Baltimore, 1987), especially pp. 57–154. Duffy, *Public Health in New York City*, pp. 307–31. A. Yankauer, "The American Journal of Public Health, 1911–85," *American Journal of Public Health* 76, no. 7 (1986): 809–15.

58 Duffy, *Public Health in New York City*, pp. 241–7, 256. Oliver, *Man Who Lived For Tomorrow*, pp. 207–12. J. Liebenau, "Public Health and the Production and Use of Diphtheria Antitoxin in Philadelphia," *Bulletin of the History of Medicine* 61, no. 2 (1987): 229, 231, 234–6. On the tension between public health organizations and physicians see J. Duffy, "The American Medical Profession and Public Health: From Support to Ambivalence," *Bulletin of the History of Medicine* 53, no. 1 (1979): 1–9.

Despite these changes in the network, the history of these years was a study primarily in cooperation across organizational and political boundaries that were still relatively permeable. The World War I experience of Mulford fits that characterization, as do the beginnings of state and federal regulation. In the decades following the dramatic changes of the 1890s, innovation in this private/public network continued, making antitoxins and vaccines more readily available to the healthcare systems in the United States and other industrialized countries. These improvements in process, in methods of distribution, and in products were less visible than the revolutionary changes of the nineties, but they were nonetheless important to the population the H. K. Mulford Company served. By the end of the 1920s, that was a substantial population indeed.

CHAPTER 3

A SHARP & DOHME INTERLUDE

T HE BALTIMORE-BASED Sharp & Dohme Company had been looking for a convenient means of moving into biologicals to extend its product line and to develop new capabilities. After the firm was reorganized in 1929, it made an offer to purchase the H. K. Mulford Company. At that time, Sharp & Dohme (S & D) was essentially a manufacturer and distributor of ethical drugs. Since its founding as a Baltimore drug store in 1845, the firm had developed new products, including for instance a "soluble hypodermic tablet" and *S.T. 37* (4-hexylresorcinol), an antiseptic solution. But in the late 1920s the company still had a very small research and development organization and had not ventured into the production of biologicals.[1] What it had done was build up an extremely effective distribution network, with branch offices in New York, Chicago, Philadelphia, Boston, Atlanta, St. Louis, New Orleans, Kansas City, Dallas, and San Francisco.[2] Lacking an R & D base or

---

1 In 1904 and 1905, Sharp & Dohme sold various serum antitoxins imported from the Pasteur Institute in Paris. These biologicals included serums for diphtheria, streptococcic infections, and tetanus. By 1906, S & D had terminated its agreement with the Pasteur Institute. See Sharp & Dohme to Dr. Walter Wyman (Surgeon General), Dec. 11, 1903, and A. R. L. Dohme to John W. Kerr (Assistant Surgeon General), Aug. 1, 1906, both in RG 90, NA. See also S & D Price-List, 1903, 1904, 1905, 1907, MA.

2 J. S. Zinsser, "Progress Through Research," address included in Sharp & Dohme, Dedication of New Medical Research Laboratories, May 12, 1952; R.

relevant production facilities upon which to build a venture into biologicals, Sharp & Dohme purchased those capabilities and looked to its own marketing organization to make the investment profitable.

The investment bankers who guided the reorganization of Sharp & Dohme and the purchase of H. K. Mulford Company quickly consolidated the two firms, bringing in new professional managers to run the business.[3] In this industry as in others, professional managers were the agents of change. They were charged with developing new organizational capabilities that would improve efficiency in the short term and position the company for success in long-term, strategic competition. When they failed, of course, they could be replaced by a new team of managers.[4]

This was what happened at Sharp & Dohme. During the early years of the Great Depression of the 1930s, the new team of managers did very little to change the Glenolden biological operations or Sharp & Dohme's other research facilities. Rather than allow that situation to continue, the firm's owners began to look for new leadership. In 1935, the Board of Directors appointed a new president, John S. Zinsser, and gave him the task of upgrading the firm's operations. As Zinsser explained: "It will be the aim of the new management to build the Company through the instrumentalities of a stricter ethical policy, more research to develop new products, and more intensified sales efforts." The new president was familiar with what companies like

Brown, "The Story of Sharp & Dohme: From Apothecary Shop to International Institution," Oct. 8, 1946; *Bulletin of the Philadelphia College of Pharmacy and Science*, Aug. 1947; E. Stauffen, "Memoir," Jan. 20, 1937; "Sharp & Dohme, Inc.," c. 1953; all in MA.

3 Frank R. Kent and Louis Azrael, *The Story of Alex Brown & Sons* (Baltimore, 1975), pp. 195–6.

4 For a discussion of the problems managers have in making these kinds of substantial, formative transitions to a new technology or science see R. S. Rosenbloom and M. Christensen, "Technological Discontinuities, Organizational Capabilities, and Strategic Commitments," *Industrial and Corporate Change* 3, no. 3 (1994): 655–85.

Merck & Co., Inc., and Eli Lilly were doing to strengthen their research capabilities, and he was determined to make Sharp & Dohme competitive.[5]

1

In the years that followed, Zinsser and his team of executives largely achieved their objectives. Before 1935, it was estimated that about 75 percent of the company's products were standard preparations sold by most of its competitors. Only 25 percent were trademarked goods. By 1951, those proportions had been reversed. Most of Sharp & Dohme's products were by that time trademarked and sold for use as directed by doctors, pharmacists, and health institutions. By 1952, when Sharp & Dohme opened a new research facility – at West Point, Pennsylvania – Zinsser could proudly announce that the firm's laboratories had "a staff of over 200 men and women, more than 70 percent of whom are scientific personnel actively engaged in the search for new and improved products for the Nation's health."[6]

But though S & D had made progress in developing its research capabilities between 1935 and 1952, most of the accomplishments were in areas other than vaccines and antitoxins. Therein lies a tale that contains some lessons – for business executives, for the political leaders who formulate policies on healthcare, and for all who are concerned about how healthcare systems perform over the long term.

While John Zinsser was attempting to build up Sharp &

---

5 Sharp & Dohme, Dedication of New Medical Research Laboratories, May 12, 1952; Hughes to Merck, Apr. 7, 1947; Sharp & Dohme, *Annual Report*, 1935; *Merck's Report*, Oct. 1929; "This is Sharp & Dohme," c. 1953; all in MA. Zinsser was a technical coordinator at Merck when he was offered the presidency of S & D. See also John Parascandola, *The Development of American Pharmacology: John J. Abel and the Shaping of a Discipline* (Baltimore, 1992), especially pp. 91–125, for the changes taking place in the company's context during these years.

6 Sharp & Dohme, Dedication of New Medical Research Laboratories, May 12, 1952; Morgan Stanley & Co., "Sharp & Dohme," c. 1950; both in MA. The company's expanded pharmaceutical manufacturing operation made use of a ball-bearing plant originally constructed for World War II production.

Since 1898 . . . This Expert Has Produced Smallpox Vaccine Mulford

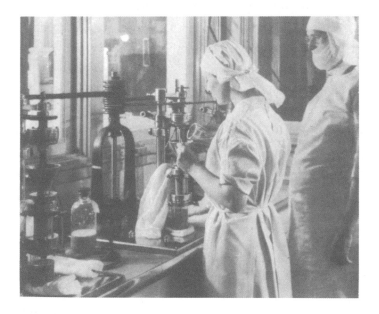

HERE Dr. William Franklin Elgin, Director of the Mulford Smallpox Vaccine Laboratory, and his assistant are grinding vaccine calf lymph. Dr. Elgin has probably made more smallpox vaccine than any other person in the world—almost one hundred millions of vaccinations since 1898! Under his direction, the Mulford Biological Laboratories have pioneered in the production of smallpox vaccine —from the old-fashioned dry ivory points, dry glass points, glycerinized glass points, to the Mulford Improved Capillary 'Tube-Points' (scarified-applicator, Mulford).

"FOR THE CONSERVATION OF LIFE"

Dohme's research and development organization, the world of medicine was being revolutionized by the discovery of anti-infectives and antibiotics. In the great rush of enthusiasm for these new drugs – for the sulfas, penicillin, and streptomycin – medical researchers everywhere turned away from vaccines and antitoxins. Why was that work needed, after all, if every infection could be treated with one of the new wonder drugs? The anti-infectives and antibiotics supplanted many of the serum antitoxins that Mulford had been producing since the turn of the century. The new drugs were more powerful and less dangerous than the serums. They seemed as well to eliminate the need for new vaccines.

So powerful were these pressures, so overblown the expectations for the new antibiotics, that during the postwar years Squibb actually abandoned two new and effective quadravalent vaccines it had developed (1944) for use against pneumococcal pneumonia. The company took this drastic action on the grounds that the vaccines simply could not be sold. Three decades later, when the need for polyvalent vaccines for pneumonia would again be recognized, Merck would receive a license for a vaccine that would protect against fourteen strains of pneumococci (covering the great majority of the serotypes that cause disease in man). But in the meantime, those scientists who decided to run counter to the trend and to continue exploring vaccinology could not always find the research positions they needed to carry on their work.[7] Companies like Sharp & Dohme also found it difficult to justify additional investments in vaccine research.

2

The worldwide quest for drug solutions was intensifying just as Sharp & Dohme was launching its effort to become a more innovative organization. President John Zinsser's training had been in chemistry and his experience at Merck had attuned him to the new developments taking

7 Chase, *Magic Shots*, pp. 26–31, 233–6; *FDA Drug Bulletin* 8, no. 1 (1978): 4–5.

place in medicinal chemistry, not to the opportunities in biologicals.[8] As a result, the company pushed ahead quickly with research on sulfonamides and new formulations of penicillin.[9] These efforts were successful, and as the wartime economy accelerated, Sharp & Dohme's sales increased between 1939 and 1948 by 252 percent. Other pharmaceutical firms, Merck included, were experiencing similar expansion. Merck's growth was based largely on its research and development efforts in vitamins and steroids, as well as antibiotics.

In biologicals, by contrast, Sharp & Dohme was not a particularly innovative organization. For most of the thirties and forties, the company was in a holding pattern, concentrating the bulk of its research efforts elsewhere.[10] Meanwhile, new investments and new personnel were needed at the firm's Glenolden biological operations, where the pace of new product development had slowed significantly during the years immediately prior to and following the merger. Aside

---

8 John S. Zinsser had an A.B. degree from Harvard University (1915) and an M.S. in Chemistry from Columbia University (1916). Following World War I, he had joined his family's chemical firm, Zinsser and Company, Inc., and had later (1934–5) worked for Merck & Co., Inc. Sharp & Dohme, Dedication of New Medical Research Laboratories, May 12, 1952, MA. Zinsser's family background was not all in chemistry; he was also related to the eminent Harvard University bacteriologist and immunologist Hans Zinsser. Haynes, *American Chemical Industry*, p. 232n.

9 For a sense of the transition that took place, compare Sharp & Dohme, Price-List, Pharmaceuticals, Biologicals, 1931 – that is, before the sulfas – with Sharp & Dohme, Price-List, Pharmaceuticals, Mulford Biologicals, Mar. 18, 1942, and Sharp & Dohme, Catalogue No. 51, May 15, 1952; all in MA. The latter price-list included numerous penicillin, sulfadiazine, sulfamerazine, sulfanilamide, sulfasuxidine (succinylsulfathiazole), sulfathalidine, sulfathiazole, and sulfonamide products.

10 Between 1930 and 1952, S & D's research staff grew from 3 to more than 200; between 1940 and 1952, research expenses (which sometimes included medical division costs) increased from $184,000 to $1,589,000. By way of comparison, Merck's research expenses had increased between 1940 and 1952 from $865,000 to $5,525,000. "Answer to FTC, Letter of July 22, 1953," MA.

from bringing out in the early 1930s a new diphtheria "toxoid" for producing active immunization and in the 1940s a vaccine for Rocky Mountain Spotted Fever,[11] Glenolden's primary function was to produce and distribute the serums, vaccines, bacterins, and serobacterins that Mulford had originally developed prior to World War I.[12] These included the successful smallpox, anthrax, and rabies vaccines; the diphtheria, tetanus, and pneumococcic serums; and a number of other biological products that would disappear from the market in the years following the Second World War.[13]

During the 1940s and early 1950s, Sharp & Dohme's major biological innovations were in blood products, especially plasma. The firm played a significant role during the Second World War in developing a new means of preserving human blood plasma. Lyophilization was a process for reducing plasma to a stable powder form that could be

---

11 Victoria A. Harden, *Rocky Mountain Spotted Fever: History of a Twentieth-Century Disease* (Baltimore, 1990), especially pp. 119–46, 175–96, 211–12, 317n. Sharp & Dohme, Price-List, Pharmaceuticals, Mulford Biologicals, Oct. 1, 1945. "Rocky Mountain Spotted Fever," in *Practical Information for Sharp & Dohme Representatives*, Jan. 1, 1947. Both in MA. The S & D product was "a chemically killed vaccine prepared from a special strain of the causative organism, Dermacentroxenus rickettsia, grown on the yolk sacs of chick embryos by the method of [Herald R.] Cox."

12 On the diphtheria toxoid see Sharp & Dohme, Price-List, Pharmaceuticals, Biologicals, 1931; Sharp & Dohme, Scientific Information, Letter No. 14, June 1, 1937 (these letters were intended to provide information to the company's sales personnel). See also the following items, all in *S & D Extract*: " 'Firsts' from Our Biological Laboratories," in 7, no. 2 (1934): 9; "The Preferred Diphtheria Prophylactic," in 3, no. 1 (1930): 2–3; and "Diphtheria Products," in 3, no. 12 (1931): 3–7. *S & D Abstract* 9, no. 2 (1936): 16–18. All in MA.

13 See *Scientific Information on Sharp & Dohme Products*, Letter No. 1, June 1, 1937, through Letter No. 51, Dec. 30, 1938. Sharp & Dohme, Pharmaceuticals, Mulford Biologicals, Oct. 1, 1945. Sharp & Dohme, Catalogue No. 51, Pharmaceuticals, Biologicals, May 15, 1952. See also the "Medical Corner," in *S & D Extract* 5, no. 5 (1933): 5–6, quoting at length from an article by Dr. Francis G. Blake, Yale University School of Medicine, providing clinical advice on serum treatment. All in MA.

Sharp & Dohme advertising stressed the high quality control standards of its Mulford laboratories.

Ampoules Are Subjected to Rigid Bacteriological Control

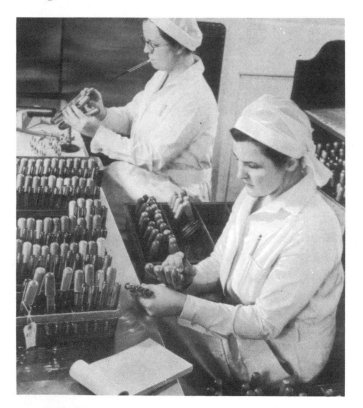

SHARP & DOHME ampoule solutions are prepared with all the care of biologicals ... with sterility established by actual test before being placed in stock. In fact, the entire filling and testing processes are conducted by our Mulford Biological Laboratories operating under government license. This includes a seven-day incubation test for sterility. A special release must be obtained from the Biological Laboratories, in addition to the approved chemical analysis of the Analytical Control Laboratory, before ampoules can be marketed. Sterility and safety are assured.

"FOR THE CONSERVATION OF LIFE"

shipped without refrigeration.[14] This dehydration technique –
involving rapid freezing and rapid dehydration under high vacuum –
would become an important means of preserving vaccines, and when
Sharp & Dohme developed a new Brucella Abortus-Strain 19 vaccine to
control brucellosis in cattle, it used this process to freeze-dry the
product.[15] But aside from that innovation, an influenza vaccine produced for the military during World War II, and a soluble antigenic
substance from *H. pertussis* (1939), the labs at Glenolden – the Mulford
Biological Laboratories of Sharp & Dohme – were not very active on
the frontiers of vaccinology.[16]

3

Those frontiers were changing in substantial ways during the 1930s
and 1940s, as a new innovative network emerged.[17] Now many of the
institutions comprising that network were national in scope. They
included the foundations that funded scientific research, as well as

---

14 E. J. Cohn, "The History of Plasma Fractionation," in U.S. Office of Scientific
Research and Development, *Advances in Military Medicine Made by American Investi-
gators Working Under the Sponsorship of the Committee on Medical Research*, ed. E. C.
Andrus, D. W. Bronk, G. A. Carden, Jr., C. S. Keefer, J. S. Lockwood, J. T.
Wearn, and M. C. Winternitz (Boston, 1948), 1:364–443.

15 Sharp & Dohme, Price-List, Pharmaceuticals, Mulford Biologicals, Oct. 1,
1945. See also "The Lyophile Technic," and "Brucella Abortus Bacterin (Heat
Killed)," in *Practical Information for Sharp & Dohme Representatives*, Jan. 1, 1947.
All in MA.

16 Compare, for instance, Sharp & Dohme, Price-List, Pharmaceuticals, Biologicals, 1931, with Sharp & Dohme, Catalogue No. 51, Pharmaceuticals, Biologicals, May 15, 1952. See also "Products of Life," June 1961; and Sharp & Dohme,
Dedication of New Medical Research Laboratories, May 12, 1952. All in MA.

17 There were of course several new "networks" evolving in medical science
during these two decades. We touch upon several of these, including the network
associated with pediatrics. For a number of years, however, the virology network
was of greatest importance to the vaccine research conducted in the private sector,
and we have thus focused most of our attention on that set of institutions and
individuals.

federal organizations such as the National Institute – later Institutes – of Health and the Centers for Disease Control.[18] America's medical education and research establishments were beginning to take leading roles in the advance of medical science; they were, in fact, just starting to shift the international flow – something comparable to an international balance of ideas – in scientific innovations. Increasingly, the freshest thinking and newest research techniques were emerging in the United States rather than Europe. Meanwhile, the new field of virology was flourishing, providing an intellectual and medical frontier comparable to the bacteriology of the 1880s and 1890s.[19]

While these developments generated significant opportunities for firms like Sharp & Dohme, the company could only take advantage of those situations if it could properly read the signals coming from this complex network and was prepared in both research and development to move ahead with promising therapies.[20] The cost of exploring this type of innovation had gone up significantly since the 1890s. It would no longer suffice to have two bacteriologists and a veterinarian working in the loft above a stable. Sharp & Dohme needed a first-class research team in biologicals: scientists who were "on the tip"; high-energy science administrators – the "brokers" who keep things moving

---

18 Robert E. Kohler, *Partners in Science: Foundations and Natural Scientists, 1900–1945* (Chicago, 1991), especially pp. 265–406. Harden, *Inventing the NIH*. Elizabeth W. Etheridge, *Sentinel for Health: A History of the Centers for Disease Control* (Berkeley, 1992).

19 A. P. Waterson and Lise Wilkinson, *An Introduction to the History of Virology* (Cambridge, Eng., 1978).

20 For discussion of these aspects of innovative organizations see L. Galambos, "The Innovative Organization: Viewed from the Shoulders of Schumpeter, Chandler, Lazonick, et al.," *Business and Economic History* 22, no. 1 (1993): 79–91; L. Galambos and J. L. Sturchio, "The Origins of an Innovative Organization: Merck & Co., Inc., 1891–1960, a Comparative Perspective" (forthcoming); and L. Galambos, "The Authority and Responsibility of the Chief Executive Officer: Shifting Patterns in Large U.S. Enterprises in the Twentieth Century," *Industrial and Corporate Change* 4, no. 1 (1995): 187–203.

in complex scientific organizations;[21] the newest equipment and facilities; and one or more "scientific diplomats," researchers or former researchers with the professional standing and political skills needed to deal with other leading institutions in this network.

Lacking these resources, Sharp & Dohme was unprepared in the 1940s and early 1950s to take full advantage of the opportunities in biologicals. Even allowing for the differences in innovation and opportunity costs, the contrast with Mulford's performance in the 1890s is telling. During the forties and fifties, Sharp & Dohme was lulled by the promise – medical and market – of the new antibiotics. Following the herd, the company remained insensitive to the significant opportunities opening up in vaccines and left itself poorly positioned to catch this next major wave of innovation. As late as 1952, when the firm's leaders recounted the organization's accomplishments and looked to the future in research, they devoted very little attention to virology and vaccines.[22]

4

At this time, neither President John Zinsser nor the company's other top executives seemed particularly attentive to the fact that Sharp & Dohme's work for the military on influenza vaccine had placed the organization on the threshold of a rapidly developing area of medical

---

21 For similar analyses of the organizational ability to read signals and to "broker" between networks and commercial organizations see Gambardella, *Science and Innovation*, especially pp. 82–105. See also N. Rosenberg, "Why Do Firms Do Basic Research (With Their Own Money)?" *Research Policy* 19, no. 2 (1990): 165–74.

22 See Sharp & Dohme, Dedication of New Medical Research Laboratories, May 12, 1952; also, Morgan Stanley & Co., "Sharp & Dohme," c. 1950; both in MA. One of the strongest arguments against a centralized system for promoting innovation over the long term is the manner in which such systems tend to adhere to dominant values and ideas, whether they come from political or professional sources. America's experience with the new antibiotics is a case in point. In this instance, progress in vaccines was certainly slowed but not stopped – as might have been true in a more centralized system. On the call for centralized, "rational" control of innovation in vaccines see Chapter 9.

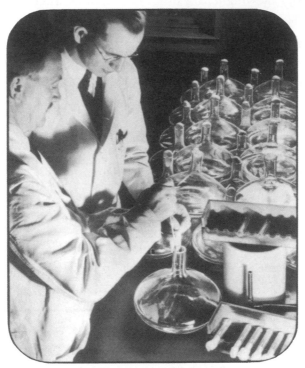

Famed "Park 8" Strain of Corynebacterium Diphtheriae . . . Used Here Since 1894

FIRST to produce Diphtheria Antitoxin commercially in the United States, the Mulford Biological Laboratories today continues to develop its diphtheria products from this famous "Park 8" strain of Corynebacterium diphtheriae.

In the illustration above, pure cultures of diphtheria bacilli are being transferred to Fernbach flasks where they grow more readily because of the larger surface. Growth takes place only on the surface, the toxin produced during growth dissolving in the medium. Later, by filtration process, all bacteria are removed, leaving the clear amber liquid which is termed diphtheria toxin.

"FOR THE CONSERVATION OF LIFE"

research. With the advantage of hindsight, we can see that Sharp & Dohme's World War II efforts on behalf of the U.S. Army were extremely important. They gave the firm experience, contacts in the network, personnel, and even an initial product – all acquired at government expense. This could have opened the door for a new strategic initiative stemming from the significant developments taking place in virology.

S & D's involvement with these scientific advances had begun after the U.S. government became concerned about the potential for an influenza epidemic. Not the least of the reasons for the Army's interest in influenza was the memory of what had happened during the great pandemic of 1918–19. Then, influenza killed between 21 and 25 million people, 549,000 of them in the United States. The military had been overwhelmed by the flu. Overcrowded conditions exacerbated the morbidity and mortality rates of this already highly contagious disease: in fact, more American men died from influenza and its secondary bacterial pneumonias in that war than were killed by the enemy. Moreover, many of the soldiers who did not die from the disease were seriously debilitated and unable to perform normal services.[23]

At that time, neither scientists nor physicians had known the source of the epidemic. Indeed, it was 1931 before medical researchers gained a significant insight into the viral cause of influenza. Then, Richard E. Shope of the Rockefeller Institute for Comparative Physiology (at Princeton), studied an apparently new disease that had emerged among swine in the early years of the twentieth century.[24] The disease

---

23 Alfred W. Crosby, Jr., *Epidemic and Peace, 1918* (Westport, CT, 1976), especially pp. 121–70; Parish, *Victory with Vaccines*, pp. 87, 162–3; Dowling, *Fighting Infection*, pp. 34, 195–8; Chase, *Magic Shots*, pp. 196–9; R. F. Betts and R. G. Douglas, "Influenza Virus," in Mandell, Douglas, and Bennett, eds., *Infectious Diseases*, p. 1306.

24 R. E. Shope, "Swine Influenza: III. Filtration Experiments and Etiology," *Journal of Experimental Medicine* 54, no. 3 (1931): 373–85. B. C. Easterday, "Animal Influenza," in Edwin D. Kilbourne, ed., *The Influenza Viruses and Influenza* (New York, 1975), pp. 449–81.

---

was swine influenza, and Shope collected a filterable virus from infected animals, introduced it to other swine, and produced the illness.

The line of research launched by Shope was soon advanced by other scientists in this new network, grounded in virology and international in scope. Scientists in England – using samples and cultures sent to them by Shope – discovered that there was a close antigenic relationship between the swine virus and the human influenza virus they had isolated. They set out to determine whether the virus collected from human throat washings could induce the disease in other animals. After many failures, they found that the disease was transferable to clean-bred ferrets and that it could be communicated back to humans from the ferrets. They discovered as well that the human sera removed from influenza convalescents conferred immunity to ferrets. They were, however, unable to develop a successful vaccine.[25]

In 1934, Dr. Thomas W. Francis at the University of Michigan confirmed the findings of the British team and also discovered antibodies in the bloodstream of animals that had convalesced from an influenza infection. The virus he isolated is now known as Type A. In 1941, Francis (then at the Hospital of the Rockefeller Institute in New York) and his former associate Thomas P. Magill at Cornell University's Influenza Strain Study Center independently isolated another influenza virus. This virus stimulated the production of antibodies that would not protect against the previously isolated influenza virus, and vice versa. That is to say, the new virus – Type B – contained different antigens. This was an important finding – one that would shape the efforts to control the disease. A successful vaccine would need to cover both serotype A and serotype B.[26]

---

25 Dowling, *Fighting Infection*, pp. 198–200; Chase, *Magic Shots*, pp. 340–3.

26 In 1950 Dr. R. M. Taylor would isolate a third strain, Type C. Dowling, *Fighting Infection*, pp. 198–200; Chase, *Magic Shots*, pp. 342–3; Betts and Douglas, "Influenza Virus," p. 1306; R. G. Douglas, Jr., "Influenza in Man," in Kilbourne, ed., *Influenza*, pp. 395–447.

Once the different strains of influenza virus had been isolated as separate disease-inducing entities, another part of this network could make important contributions. Epidemiologists – many of them connected to the growing public health system – could now study to useful effect the different outbreaks. As of 1947 when the World Health Organization established a system of collaborating laboratories, this part of the network was also international in scope.[27] As became apparent, each type had a specific pattern in terms of the cyclic nature and frequency of epidemics and the severity of the illness. Type A virus, for example, was found to cause major epidemics every two to three years, whereas the milder epidemics associated with Type B virus erupted every three to six years.[28]

5

It was at this point that the focus of research shifted to another set of public institutions, the military. During the war, the U.S. Army's special commission on influenza and other epidemic diseases (later, the Army Epidemiological Board) sponsored research conducted by Dr. Francis and his colleagues. In 1943, with the help of Fred Davenport and Jonas Salk, Francis produced a formalin-inactivated influenza vaccine for the military. This was an important step toward providing immunity because this vaccine conferred substantial protection for as much as six months. The success of the vaccine encouraged the U.S. Army to contract with Sharp & Dohme and several other manufactur-

---

27 M. S. Pereira, "Strain Surveillance in Man," in Philip Selby, ed., *Influenza: Virus, Vaccines, and Strategy* (New York, 1976), pp. 25–31. World Health Organization, Expert Committee on Influenza, "First Report," *World Health Organization Technical Report Series* 64 (1953). On the state of epidemiology see Chapin, *State Public Health Work*, pp. 118–20; Fee, *Disease and Discovery*, pp. 68–70, 132–6, 161–2; and Etheridge, *Sentinel for Health*, pp. 39–48.

28 Betts and Douglas, "Influenza Virus," pp. 1310–12; Dowling, *Fighting Infection*, p. 199.

ers with biological capabilities to begin to produce the vaccine for military use.[29]

Moving from the laboratory to the production line proved to be a major problem. The science was of recent vintage and as yet rudimentary; biological manufacturing had in recent years been a static area of pharmaceutical development. Sharp & Dohme grew the virus in the allantoic sacs of embryonated hens' eggs and purified it by adsorption to and elution from red blood cells. The virus was inactivated by treatment with formaldehyde. Several aspects of the process were labor intensive and the product was crude by present-day standards. Working under wartime pressure, Sharp & Dohme was able to supply the Army with 20,000 shots of a bivalent (Type A plus Type B), killed-virus vaccine.[30] The vaccine was used successfully during an epidemic in 1944, and the following year the government licensed Sharp & Dohme to produce and sell the product for civilian use.[31]

During and immediately after the war, Sharp & Dohme began to utilize and to develop a number of process innovations in its vaccine program. The company was able now to do a quantitative assay for the amount of virus to include in the vaccine by using the chick cell agglutination (CCA) test, a process that greatly simplified the task of measuring the strength of the vaccine. Later, when the company began mass production, it devised special syringes to inoculate the embryonated eggs, developed new techniques for candling the eggs to eliminate those that were infertile or in which the embryos had died, and invented a new instrument for harvesting the infected egg allantoic fluid.

All that was lacking was commercial success. The new influ-

---

29 U.S. Army Medical Service, *Preventive Medicine in World War II*, vol. 3, *Personal Health Measures and Immunization*, ed. John Boyd Coates, Jr., Ebbe Curtis Hoff, and Phebe M. Hoff (Washington, DC, 1955), pp. 323–7.

30 S & D purified the influenza virus by protamine precipitation.

31 R. C. Bostwick to Robert L. Banse, et al., Dec. 3, 1971, with enclosed lists of licensed products, MA.

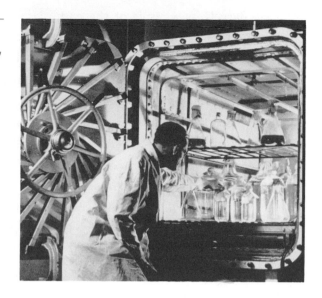

*Sharp & Dohme's
biological laboratory
in the 1930s.*

enza vaccine did not sell very well. It was not widely used because it afforded only temporary immunity and had to be injected. The major problem, however, was its reactogenicity. The shots frequently caused such sore arms and fevers that patients had every reason to conclude that it would have been better to take their chances with the flu.[32] Based on this experience alone, virology still did not seem to Sharp & Dohme's executives to justify much additional attention or capital investment.

6

By the early 1950s, when Sharp & Dohme dedicated its extensive new research facilities at West Point, Pennsylvania, the firm's experience with the fast-developing field of virology had not been particularly successful, either commercially or scientifically. Throughout the industry, new product development in vaccines and serums had virtually

32 U.S. Army Medical Service, *Preventive Medicine*, 3:326–7. June E. Osborn, ed., *History, Science, and Politics: Influenza in America, 1918–1976* (New York, 1977), pp. 17–18. Harvard Business School, "Merck & Co., Inc." (Case Study, 1960). The reactogenicity was a product of the relative impurity of the vaccine, a problem that was not solved until the 1960s.

stopped, largely as a result of the enthusiasm for antibiotics. This interlude in the industry's development provided a good rationale for having a decentralized, mixed system in which neither markets nor political authority could completely dominate the professional factors shaping science and technology. The science of virology, responding to different incentives, continued to evolve in fruitful ways despite the absence of support from the industry or the government.

Meanwhile, S & D was continuing to market a full line of biologicals for human and veterinary use. Most of these products had been introduced by the Glenolden laboratories before 1929 and many of them before 1919. Sharp & Dohme had acquired Mulford with two strategic objectives in mind, only one of which had been achieved. Sharp & Dohme had indeed broadened its product line; but it had not developed an organization with substantial capability for innovation in biologicals. The opportunities were growing, but the firm was not yet equipped to take advantage of them.

Like other companies in the industry, Sharp & Dohme was watching from the sidelines the network of research institutions and new ideas that would revolutionize both virology and vaccinology in the postwar years. Vaccine development stood at the threshhold of an era characterized by "a better science made possible by the development of a sophisticated cell culture technology and the origination of usefully applied subunit polysaccharide vaccines against certain of the gram positive and gram negative cocci."[33] The discovery of how DNA governs the cell and the development of the electron microscope would transform immunology and virology. The electron microscope would do for virology what the bench microscope had done for bacteriology. Now researchers could for the first time actually see the viruses with which they were working.

But before Sharp & Dohme could establish close links with these important developments, the firm would need to make a substan-

---

33 M. R. Hilleman, "The Science of Vaccines in Present and Future Perspective," *Medical Journal of Australia* 144 (Mar. 31, 1986): 360–4.

tial investment in biological research. It is understandable why Sharp & Dohme had not made those investments during the 1930s, when the national economy was experiencing the worst depression in its history; this decision is less understandable in the immediate postwar years, when profits were higher and economic opportunities for U.S. firms in these industries were growing. Then, the laboratory's biological team was still small and oriented primarily to medical chemistry and pharmacology. While the company's virology department included eleven researchers, only four of them had doctorates and none was an international leader in the new science.[34]

It is not at all clear that Sharp & Dohme had the scale to afford innovation in more than one line of biologicals. In the 1940s and 1950s, it had invested in biological innovation involving blood products, a market greatly expanded by the war effort. There appear to have been very few economies of scope between the serum research and the research on antitoxins and vaccines. The new developments in virology called for an in-house level of scientific expertise much higher than anything Sharp & Dohme had achieved prior to 1953. It called as well for a long-term strategic commitment to the transfer of company resources from the relatively predictable antibiotics and blood products to a higher-risk undertaking in vaccines. The firm's executives were not prepared to make that commitment. Shortly, those conditions would change following a merger that transformed Sharp & Dohme, its new partner, Merck & Co., Inc., and indeed the global pharmaceutical and biologicals industries.

---

34 The personnel and their degrees are listed in Sharp & Dohme, Dedication of New Medical Research Laboratories, May 12, 1952, MA.

CHAPTER 4

THE VIROLOGY NETWORK AND A NEW
PROGRAM AT MERCK SHARP & DOHME

F OR THE biologicals and pharmaceutical industries of the United States, the decades following World War II were filled with unusual opportunities. In the domestic economy, these were years of prosperity and growth, labeled "The American Century" by *Life* magazine's Henry Luce. As that slogan correctly predicted, the United States emerged from the war as the world's dominant economic power, and the nation's multinational corporations were now able to penetrate foreign markets that had long been controlled by European and Asian competitors.[1] Economies of scale and scope were important sources of competitive advantage.[2] But the growth of U.S. companies was also propelled by the innovations stemming from their fruitful interaction

---

1 Angus Maddison, *Economic Growth in the West: Comparative Experience in Europe and North America* (New York, 1964), especially pp. 43–98. The same author's *Dynamic Forces in Capitalist Development* (New York, 1991). L. Hannah, "Delusions of Durable Dominance or the Invisible Hand Strikes Back" (draft manuscript, courtesy of the author, 1995). Louis Galambos and Joseph Pratt, *The Rise of the Corporate Commonwealth: U.S. Business and Public Policy in the Twentieth Century* (New York, 1988), pp. 127–83.

2 Chandler, *Scale and Scope*; and Alfred D. Chandler, Jr., and Herman Daems, *Managerial Hierarchies: Comparative Perspectives on the Rise of the Modern Industrial Enterprise* (Cambridge, MA, 1980).

with America's complex array of professions, including those in science and engineering.[3]

Science-based industries benefited from the burgeoning of a new government/university complex that pumped billions of public dollars into professional training and research. Many of the federal programs were justified by reference to national security and all were buttressed by the widespread confidence that the nation's success in World War II had to a considerable degree been a product of its scientific and technological prowess.[4] In this favorable economic and political setting, complex innovative networks developed in electronic computing, atomic power, microwave transmission, liquid gases, medicinal chemistry, biochemistry, and virology – to mention only a few.[5] In the fields related to medical science, the national security theme was *sotto voce*, and this facilitated the exchange of ideas nationally and internationally. As we have seen, cooperative exchanges of this sort had been extremely fruitful for America and for its medical sciences

---

3 John W. Kendrick, *Productivity in the United States: Trends and Cycles* (Baltimore, 1980). Edward F. Denison, *Accounting for United States Economic Growth, 1929–1969* (Washington, DC, 1974). M. Abramovitz and P. A. David, "Reinterpreting Economic Growth: Parables and Realities," *American Economic Review* 63, no. 2 (1973): 428–39. Simon S. Kuznets, *Modern Economic Growth: Rate, Structure and Spread* (New Haven, 1966).

4 Stuart W. Leslie, *The Cold War and American Science: The Military-Industrial-Academic Complex at MIT and Stanford* (New York, 1993). See also the carefully researched survey by P. Forman, "Behind Quantum Electronics: National Security as Basis for Physical Research in the United States, 1940–1960," *Historical Studies in the Physical and Biological Sciences* 18, no. 1 (1987): 149–229.

5 Forman, "Behind Quantum Electronics," pp. 149–229. On the development of the transistor see T. J. Misa, "Military Needs, Commercial Realities, and the Development of the Transistor, 1948–1958," in Merritt Roe Smith, *Military Enterprise and Technological Change: Perspectives on the American Experience* (Cambridge, MA, 1987), pp. 251–87. On atomic energy see Brian Balogh, *Chain Reaction: Expert Debate and Public Participation in American Commercial Nuclear Power, 1945–1975* (New York, 1991).

---

during the earlier cycle of innovation in which the H. K. Mulford Company had been an active participant.

Of course all of the new institutional relationships of "The American Century" were not conducive to cooperation and innovation. As the regulatory setting in the United States became more elaborate and relationships more adversarial, firms in pharmaceuticals and biologicals, for example, found it necessary to invest more time, money, and expertise in dealing with organizations like the Food and Drug Administration (FDA) and the Division of Biologics Standards.[6] In vaccine development, a series of crises strained public-private ties, prompting the administrative state to tighten its controls. Over the years, lines of communication became more bureaucratic and boundaries between institutions more formal. In the public and nonprofit spheres, competition for resources and recognition became at times something akin to business competition for market shares, and this too had a negative impact on the innovative process.

While the division of the postwar world into communist and noncommunist blocs frequently undercut cooperation across national frontiers, the main thrust of institutional change in these years was toward internationalism. Transportation and communications improvements fostered this development, as did the increasing role of multinational firms in business. A number of new or refurbished institutions – including the United Nations, the World Health Organization, the Pan American Health Organization, and the World Bank Group – came to play important roles in the efforts during these years to im-

---

6 E. J. Jensen, "Research Expenditures and the Discovery of New Drugs," *Journal of Industrial Economics* 36, no. 1 (1987): 93–4. Henry G. Grabowski, *Drug Regulation and Innovation: Empirical Evidence and Policy Options* (Washington, DC, 1976). Henry G. Grabowski and John M. Vernon, *The Regulation of Pharmaceuticals: Balancing the Benefits and Risks* (Washington, DC, 1983). J. M. Vernon and P. Gusen, "Technical Change and Firm Size: The Pharmaceutical Industry," *Review of Economics and Statistics* 56, no. 3 (1977): 294–302. L. G. Thomas, "Regulation and Firm Size: FDA Impacts on Innovation," *Rand Journal of Economics* 21, no. 4 (1990): 497–517.

prove immunization levels and upgrade other aspects of healthcare throughout the world.[7]

1

In this challenging environment, private firms like Sharp & Dohme and Merck & Co., Inc., had to develop new capabilities if they were going to succeed. By 1953, Merck was one of the nation's leading producers of fine chemicals and pharmaceuticals. This Rahway, New Jersey manufacturing firm had one of the world's premier research and development organizations in medicinal chemistry, and its laboratories, pilot plants, and factories had since the 1930s played a central role in the development of synthetic vitamins, antibiotics, anti-infectives, and steroids.[8] It was, nevertheless, an organization facing an uncertain future by the early 1950s. It sold most of its products to other firms – including Sharp &

---

7 See June Goodfield, *A Chance to Live* (New York, 1991), pp. 25–42. P. Dorolle, "Old Plagues in the Jet Age: International Aspects of Present and Future Control of Communicable Diseases," *World Health Organization Chronicle* 23 (1969): 103–11. *The World Health Organization* (Geneva, c. 1967). Norman Howard-Jones, *The Pan American Health Organization: Origins and Evolution* (Geneva, 1981). Pan American Health Organization, *The Crisis of Public Health: Reflections for the Debate* (Washington, DC, 1992), especially pp. 121–33, 166–83.

8 On Merck's role in synthetic vitamins see "Vitamins" (manuscript, Merck & Co., Inc., 1959), MA. On anti-infectives and antibiotics see: W. H. Helfand, H. B. Woodruff, K. M. M. Coleman, and D. L. Cowen, "Wartime Industrial Development of Penicillin in the United States," in John Parascandola, ed., *A History of Antibiotics* (Madison, WI, 1980), pp. 31–56. J. L. Sturchio, "Chemistry in Action: Penicillin Production in World War II," *Today's Chemist* 1, no. 1 (1988): 20–2, 35–6. M. Tishler, "Production and Isolation of Streptomycin," in Selman A. Waksman, ed., *Streptomycin: Nature and Practical Applications* (Baltimore, 1949), pp. 32–54. On steroids see: "A Progress Report on Cortisone: Key to a New Era of Medical Science," (1950); and R. T. Major, "Cortisone – A Product of Joint Academic and Industrial Research" (n.d.); both in MA. See also L. Galambos and J. L. Sturchio, "The Origins of an Innovative Organization: Merck & Co., Inc., 1891–1960" (paper presented to the Society for the History of Technology, Aug. 1992), pp. 14–29. And Jeffrey L. Sturchio, ed., *Values and Visions: A Merck Century* (Rahway, NJ, 1991), especially pp. 65–81.

Dohme – that turned the materials into finished pharmaceuticals. But increasingly Merck's customers were integrating backward into the production of their own supplies. Merck could of course counter this strategy by making its own trademarked drugs, but it lacked an effective marketing organization to sell the finished products.[9] It needed a partner, an established pharmaceutical company with the sales representatives and distribution system that would enable Merck to take its products to the "customers": the doctors and health establishments that controlled the market for prescription drugs.

Sharp & Dohme was thus an ideal partner for Merck. A longtime customer of the Rahway firm, Sharp & Dohme was led by two officers who were former Merck employees and who knew the chemical firm's strengths. With their assistance, Merck completed the merger in 1953 – although it took considerably longer than that to integrate the two organizations' operations. While there is some evidence that the process of integration is still going on today, administrative consolidation in research accelerated sharply after Merck centralized all of R & D under the Merck Sharp & Dohme Research Laboratories (MSDRL, 1956) and appointed Dr. Max Tishler as president of that organization the following year.[10]

By that time, Merck had also made a decisive move into

---

9 O. H. Schell, Jr., Memorandum, Nov. 17, 1947; "Vitamins," Nov. 1959; Mr. Green to Mr. Merck, Nov. 17, 1947; J. T. Connor, "The Merck-Sharp & Dohme Merger," Oct. 13, 1954; all in MA.

10 Tishler was an outstanding organic chemist who had left Harvard University to join Merck in 1937. Max Tishler, Oral History, July 13, 1988, MA. On the reorganization of scientific activities see the following: A. N. Richards to V. Bush, Mar. 29, 1952; V. Bush to A. N. Richards, Mar. 31 and Nov. 12, 1952; V. Bush to J. J. Kerrigan, Mar. 24, 1954; J. T. Connor to G. W. Merck, May 13, 1954; Office of the Secretary to Management Council, Aug. 24, 1955; A. N. Richards to V. Bush, Jan. 22, 1955; and V. Bush to A. N. Richards, Feb. 10, 1955; all in Bush Papers, Library of Congress, hereafter LC. Also see R. T. Major to J. J. Kerrigan, June 22, 1955; and A. N. Richards to V. Bush, Aug. 14, 1955; in A. N. Richards Papers, University of Pennsylvania Archives, hereafter UPA.

international operations. Using as its base the Sharp & Dohme overseas distribution network, Merck began to establish a series of subsidiaries in Latin America and Europe. It also strengthened its ties with Banyu, a Japanese pharmaceutical company.[11] Led by a fresh cadre of professional managers, Merck was a growing business that looked to MSDRL for the innovative pharmaceuticals and biologicals it needed to sustain its expansion. In the 1950s the firm made a fundamental strategic decision to stop active promotion and sometimes production of products – as it did vitamins – when they became generics. In effect, that bet the company's future on the ability of the laboratories to continue to develop new drugs for which there would be substantial markets at home and abroad. The capacity for successful innovation became the central element in Merck's corporate strategy from the 1950s on – and is still the lynchpin of its strategy today.

Little wonder then that the new president of MSDRL (Merck Sharp & Dohme Research Laboratories) and the firm's other leaders began to look with a critical eye at their biological research organization. Since 1956, when the firm sold the Glenolden properties, all of the research in biologicals had been concentrated at West Point, Pennsylvania.[12] There, the firm had research teams working on veterinary vaccines and on a vaccine for polio.[13]

---

11 J. H. Sharp to J. T. Connor, "Interim Report of Task Force for Foreign Field," July 13, 1953; "Transcript of the Presentations to the Board of Directors of Merck & Co., Inc.," Oct. 26, 1972; "MSDI On The Move!" *Merck Review* 23, no. 2 (1962); all in MA. J. H. Sharp to Board of Directors, Nov. 23, 1954; and Organization of Merck Sharp & Dohme International Division of Merck & Co., Inc., May 11, 1955; in Bush Papers, LC.

12 Max Tishler, Oral History, July 13, 1988, MA. Scientific Coordinating Committee Meeting, Dec. 16, 1954, Bush Papers, LC. See also "Some Thoughts About Merck Institute," Major to Kerrigan, June 22, 1955, and Arnow to Richards and Major, Sept. 21, 1953; all in Richards Papers, UPA.

13 For more extensive reviews see "Scientific Area – Medical Division, Proposed Program," Mar. 11, 1955; and "Report to the Scientific Advisors of the Merck Institute," June 10, 1957; in UPA.

Research in the United States on polio had been greatly accelerated after Dr. John F. Enders and his coworkers at the Children's Hospital in Boston discovered that they could grow the virus in human and monkey tissue cultures and could directly observe and measure its cytopathic effects. This and Enders's other innovations in tissue culture provided one of the foundation stones of modern virology, a field of medical science that was in the 1950s creating significant opportunities for firms like Merck to develop new commercial products.[14]

The tissue culture innovations of Enders, et al., prompted an experiment in cooperative technical research guided by a committee. Much in the style of the large wartime projects, the undertaking sponsored in the early 1950s by the Technical Committee of the National Foundation for Infantile Paralysis had the goal of developing a killed-virus vaccine for polio.[15] The committee members contracted to work on discrete aspects of the technical problems involved and Dr. Jonas Salk and his associates at the University of Pittsburgh were assigned the job of growing the virus *en masse*, inactivating it, and conducting tests for potency and safety. By 1954 this coordinated effort had produced a killed-polio-virus vaccine that was effective against all three serotypes of the virus and that appeared to be ready for use in a large-scale national test.[16]

---

14 Chase, *Magic Shots*, pp. 286–301. J. F. Enders, T. H. Weller, and F. C. Robbins, "Cultivation of the Lansing Strain of Poliomyelitis Virus in Cultures of Various Human Embryonic Tissue," *Science* 109 (Jan. 28, 1949): 85. R. Ward, "Poliomyelitis," *Symposium on Infectious Diseases* 7, no. 4 (1960), especially pp. 960–2.

15 The primary difference between the polio campaign and the wartime ventures was that the polio effort was coordinated by a private foundation and not by the federal government. In that sense, it represented a transitional phase between the interwar institutional networks and those of the post-World War II era. On this transition see Kohler, *Partners in Science*.

16 Jane E. Smith, *Patenting the Sun: Polio and the Salk Vaccine* (New York, 1990), provides a useful narrative; see especially pp. 109–369. See also Aaron E. Klein, *Trial By Fury: The Polio Vaccine Controversy* (New York, 1972); and Richard Carter,

Just as this particular network of public and private institutions was on the edge of success, however, a number of problems developed. Some of them stemmed from the politicization of the processes of discovery and delivery. Others resulted from the lack of knowledge on this scientific frontier. Whatever the cause, a number of firms in biologicals became entangled in the ensuing difficulties.[17] Merck's laboratory at West Point was one of those commissioned to produce vaccine for the experimental program, but Dr. Betty Lee Hampil, who was in charge of virology at West Point, decided she could not release the company's vaccine. She had discovered in one of her tests that brain lesions had formed in monkeys when larger amounts of the vaccine were injected than the FDA had specified. She had concerns about safety if the virus was not entirely inactivated. The history of vaccine development for this disease favored caution despite the intense public pressure to accelerate the tests. In the 1930s, two earlier polio vaccines had been given clinical tests and then withdrawn after a number of those receiving the shots had developed polio and died.[18]

The firm's executives agreed with Hampil and left Merck on

Breakthrough: The Saga of Jonas Salk (New York, 1965), two popular accounts. We have given less emphasis here to Dr. Jonas Salk than do most accounts of these events. Although Salk's contribution was important and was appropriately acknowledged, this project involved a well organized team effort, and we think appropriate recognition should also be given to the work of Drs. Thomas Francis, Howard H. Howe, Joseph Smadel, David Bodian, and William McDowell Hammon, among others.

17 The ethical issues are explored in A. M. Brandt, "Polio, Politics, Publicity, and Duplicity: Ethical Aspects in the Development of the Salk Vaccine," *Connecticut Medicine* 43, no. 9 (1979): 581–90. See also B. Spector, "The Great Salk Vaccine Mess," *Antioch Review* (1980): 291–303.

18 L. B. Berk, "Polio Vaccine Trials of 1935," *Transactions and Studies of the College of Physicians of Philadelphia*, 5th ser., 11, no. 4 (1989): 321–36. See also John R. Paul, *A History of Poliomyelitis* (New Haven, CT, 1971), pp. 252–62. But for a different interpretation of the failure see H. V. Wyatt, "Provocation Poliomyelitis: Neglected Clinical Observations from 1914 to 1950," *Bulletin of the History of Medicine* 55, no. 4 (1981): 543–57.

the sidelines as the highly publicized national test proceeded.[19] Although the company had experienced public and governmental pressure before – during World War II, for instance, when it played a leading role in penicillin development and production – this was a far more intense experience. The national media was aquiver and the vibrations from the press kept Washington, D.C., on full alert. Then, just as the favorable results from the national test were being released, tragedy struck. Some of the batches of vaccine from the Cutter Laboratories contained live virus and 260 cases of polio and eleven deaths would be traced to Cutter's vaccine.[20]

Although the polio campaign survived this early crisis, the Cutter incident revealed how much had changed in this emerging network of national institutions and immunization programs. Private firms like Merck had every reason to be extremely cautious about providing the vaccines that would be injected into millions of apparently healthy children. The government purchased and administered the vaccines. But the private companies were liable for damages, even if they closely adhered to the prescribed procedures and gave adequate warning about the possible dangers of vaccination. Any private corporation producing vaccines had to ask whether the increased liability and the narrower profit margins resulting from large-scale government purchasing did not outweigh the opportunities generated by the new setting.[21]

19 Max Tishler, Oral History, July 13, 1988, MA.

20 Chase, *Magic Shots*, p. 298. A number of scientists had reservations about the Salk killed-virus vaccine, and the Laboratory of Biologics Control had reservations about the vaccines produced by several of the manufacturers. But the public pressure to move ahead with the tests was extremely strong. Brandt, "Polio, Politics," p. 584. See also Paul, *History of Poliomyelitis*, pp. 435–8.

21 It would be 1986 before Congress would pass and President Ronald Reagan sign into law the National Childhood Vaccine Injury Act. The law would provide for no-fault government compensation for injuries stemming from *existing* pediatric vaccines. J. K. Iglehart, "Health Policy Report: Compensating Children with Vaccine-Related Injuries," *New England Journal of Medicine* 316, no. 20 (1987):

In the years ahead, many companies in biologicals would decide that the risks outweighed the opportunities, but Merck executives came to the opposite conclusion. The Merck Sharp and Dohme Research Laboratories continued research on polio vaccine and the firm for a limited time became a major supplier.[22] But that took place under a new research team organized in an effort to give Merck a leadership position in this new network and its related markets.

2

Max Tishler, the new president of MSDRL, decided that if the company was going to stay in biologicals it needed to build up its research program in virology and vaccines. The transformation in research had to be formative, not incremental.[23] Tishler's own background was in organic chemistry and most of his innovations at Merck since the 1930s had involved improvements in processes, on the development side of R & D. But Tishler appreciated what was happening in virology, and he had strong support for a forceful strategic move in this direction. Vannevar Bush, chairman of Merck's Board, was convinced that the firm should become a leader in this area of research, and Bush was an effective advocate for any strategic

---

1283–8. See also "HRSA Proposes Changes in Vaccine Injury Compensation Program," *Public Health Reports* 107, no. 6 (1992): 741.

22 Merck Sharp & Dohme would deliver its first shipment of Salk polio vaccine on May 21, 1956. The firm planned to reach full production by the fall of that year. *MSD Sales Dispatch* 116 (June 1956); 125 (Apr. 1957); in MA.

23 In the language of current research-policy analysis, Tishler wanted "architectural," not incremental, change. R. M. Henderson and K. B. Clark, "Architectural Innovation: The Reconfiguration of Existing Product Technologies and the Failure of Established Firms," *Administrative Science Quarterly* 35, no. 1 (1990): 9–30. We have used instead the language of business history to make the same distinction. See William Lazonick, *Business Organization and the Myth of the Market Economy* (New York, 1991), especially pp. 198–227. L. Galambos, "The Innovative Organization: Viewed from the Shoulders of Schumpeter, Chandler, Lazonick, et al.," *Business and Economic History* 22, no. 1 (1993): 79–91.

decision he favored.[24] In this case, he had the support of Merck's longtime scientific advisor, Dr. Alfred Newton Richards. Merck's CEO, John Connor, was also enthusiastic about this strategic initiative, as was the firm's chief operating officer, President Henry Gadsden.[25] Both were willing by 1956–7 to provide Tishler with the resources he would need.[26]

---

24 For background on Bush see N. Reingold, "Vannevar Bush's New Deal for Research: Or the Triumph of the Old Order," *Historical Studies in the Physical and Biological Sciences* 17, no. 2 (1987): 299–344. On Bush and the Merck board of directors see L. Galambos and J. L. Sturchio, "Origins of an Innovative Organization," pp. 27–8; see also the considerable body of correspondence between Bush and Merck in the Bush Papers, LC.

25 John T. Connor received his B.A. from Syracuse University in 1936 and his LL.B. from the Harvard Law School in 1939. After working for three years at a New York City law firm, he went to the Office of Scientific Research and Development (Washington, DC), where he was general counsel (1942–4). Following service with the Marine Corps in the Pacific Theatre, he returned to Washington, to the Office of Naval Research. He was counsel and then special assistant to Secretary of the Navy James Forrestal (1945–7). He joined Merck as a general attorney in 1947 and was successively secretary, counsel, and vice president of the company. He was Merck's president from 1955 to 1965, when he retired to become secretary of commerce under President Lyndon B. Johnson.

26 Max Tishler, Oral History, July 13, 1988, MA. We have also had the benefit of extensive handwritten notes by Dr. Maurice R. Hilleman, who read and commented on an early draft of this manuscript; Hilleman provided us with Tishler's contemporary explanation of this decision. M. R. Hilleman, "Notes," MA. See John T. Connor, Interview, Dec. 27, 1991, for a third version of the decision. See also L. E. Arnow, Report of the Executive Director to the Board of Trustees of the Merck Institute for Therapeutic Research, Feb. 1, 1957, Richards Papers, UPA.

For an indication of how much changed when Tishler took over at MSDRL, compare Arnow's statement, "We are searching actively for a virologist of stature to headup our program in virology" (ibid.), with the record of the Scientific Coordinating Committee Meeting, Dec. 16, 1954, and R. T. Major to J. J. Kerrigan, Mar. 21, 1955, both in Bush Papers, LC. Neither of the latter documents indicated that major changes were needed at that time in virology.

But to implement that strategy, Tishler first had to locate a world-class virologist who was willing to reconceptualize, reorganize, and restaff the West Point operation. More was involved with this position than laboratory science. Betty Lee Hampil was nearing retirement, and besides, she was not the sort of scientific diplomat who could give the firm a central role in this rapidly evolving area of medical science. The experience with the Salk trials had been revealing.[27] The new institutional setting for vaccine development and distribution was extremely complex and was national and increasingly international in scope. It was supercharged with media attention and political pressure and was sprinkled with legal and regulatory mine fields for a commercial enterprise. What Merck needed if it was going to occupy a central role in this network was a leader who was "a great scientist *and* a great mover."[28]

Fortunately for Tishler, a scientist who had these qualifications had been working with Merck as a consultant.[29] Unfortunately for Tishler, it was not at all clear that Dr. Maurice R. Hilleman would leave his position as chief of the Department of Respiratory Diseases at the Walter Reed Army Institute of Research in Washington, D.C. The Institute at Walter Reed was a major center for research in virology, and Hilleman had spent ten highly productive years there under the

---

27 After launching its tissue culture and polio research, Merck had attempted (unsuccessfully) to hire Jonas Salk as a consultant. Max Tishler, Oral History, July 13, 1988, MA. Smith, *Patenting the Sun*, pp. 217–18. Prior to the merger with Sharp & Dohme, Merck had employed Dr. Richard E. Shope as an assistant director of the Merck Institute (1949–52). Shope had helped the Institute establish its tissue culture research, but he had found "work within a commercial organization was quite foreign to his temperament" and had returned to New York to the Rockefeller University. C. Andrewes, "Richard Edwin Shope, December 25, 1901–October 2, 1966," in National Academy of Sciences, *Biographical Memoirs* (Washington, DC, 1979), 50:362. John T. Connor, Interview, Dec. 27, 1988.

28 Max Tishler, Oral History, July 13, 1988, MA. Emphasis added.

29 Maurice R. Hilleman, Interview, Nov. 13 and 21, 1991.

An emergency shipment of Merck Sharp & Dohme vaccine in 1956.

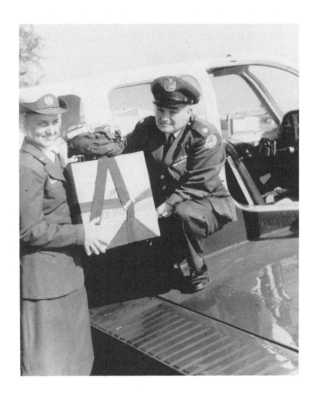

tutelage of Dr. Joseph Smadel, who headed the Division of Communicable Diseases.[30]

During those years, Hilleman had been a codiscoverer of the respiratory viruses now known as adenoviruses, had developed diagnostic tests for and defined the clinical features of the diseases caused by three of the viruses, and had produced an effective killed-virus vaccine.[31] In addition to this breakthrough in pediatric and military

---

30 Hilleman later characterized Smadel as a "charismatic genius." M. R. Hilleman, "Notes," MA.

31 M. R. Hilleman and J. H. Werner, "Recovery of New Agent from Patients with Acute Respiratory Illness," *Proceedings of the Society for Experimental Biology and Medicine* 85 (1954): 183–8; M. R. Hilleman, J. H. Werner, H. E. Dascomb, and R. L. Butler, "Epidemiological Investigations with Respiratory Disease Virus RI-67," *American Journal of Public Health* 45, no. 2 (1955): 203–10; M. R. Hilleman, J. H. Werner, C. V. Adair, and A. R. Dreisbach, "Outbreak of Acute

medicine, Hilleman had done work of fundamental importance on shift and drift in the antigenic form of influenza viruses.[32] During his tenure, Walter Reed had become a major center for the study of influenza epidemiology by use of virus strain analysis and retrospective seroepidemiology. Although diplomatic discourse was not Hilleman's common mode of communication, he was qualified by

Respiratory Illness Caused by RI-67 and Influenza A Viruses, Fort Leonard Wood, 1952–1953," *American Journal of Hygiene* 61, no. 2 (1955): 163–73; M. R. Hilleman, J. H. Werner, and M. T. Stewart, "Grouping and Occurrence of RI (Prototype RI-67) Viruses," *Proceedings of the Society for Experimental Biology and Medicine* 90 (1955): 555–62; M. R. Hilleman, A. J. Tousimis, and J. H. Werner, "Biophysical Characterization of RI (RI-67) Viruses," *Proceedings of the Society for Experimental Biology and Medicine* 89 (1955): 587–93; M. R. Hilleman, J. H. Werner, H. E. Dascomb, R. L. Butler, and M. T. Stewart, "Epidemiology of RI (RI-67) Group Respiratory Virus Infections in Recruit Populations," *American Journal of Hygiene* 62, no. 1 (1955): 29–43; C. M. Southam, M. R. Hilleman, and J. H. Werner, "Pathogenicity and Oncolytic Capacity of RI Virus Strain RI-67 in Man," *Journal of Laboratory and Clinical Medicine* 47, no. 4 (1956): 573–82; H. E. Dascomb and M. R. Hilleman, "Clinical and Laboratory Studies in Patients with Respiratory Disease Caused by Adenoviruses (RI-APC-ARD Agents)," *American Journal of Medicine* 21, no. 2 (1956): 161–74; J. F. Enders, J. A. Bell, J. H. Dingle, T. Francis, Jr., and M. R. Hilleman, " 'Adenoviruses': Group Name Proposed for New Respiratory Tract Viruses," *Science* 124 (July 20, 1956): 119–20.

32 M. R. Hilleman, R. P. Mason, and E. L. Buescher, "Antigenic Pattern of Strains of Influenza A and B," *Proceedings of the Society for Experimental Biology and Medicine* 75 (1950): 829–35; M. R. Hilleman, "System for Measuring and Designating Antigenic Components of Influenza Viruses with Analyses of Recently Isolated Strains," *Proceedings of the Society for Experimental Biology and Medicine* 78 (1951): 208–15; M. R. Hilleman, "A Pattern of Antigen Variation," American Association of Immunologists' Symposium on Antigenic Variation of Influenza Viruses and Its Importance in Vaccination, *Federation Proceedings* 11 (1952): 798–803; M. R. Hilleman, J. H. Werner, and R. L. Gauld, "Serological Studies of Influenza Antibodies in the Population of the United States: An Epidemiological Investigation," *Bulletin of the World Health Organization* 8 (1953): 613–31; M. R. Hilleman, "Antigenic Variation of Influenza Viruses," *Annual Review of Microbiology* 8 (1954): 311–32.

experience and temperament to play the special role – inside the firm and outside – that Tishler and the other Merck officers had in mind. Tishler and Connor were convinced that in addition to being "a great scientist," he was the "great mover" they needed.[33]

Hilleman was certainly an imposing and to some even an intimidating figure, with a long track record of scientific successes. Reared outside of tiny Miles City, Montana, Hilleman had spent his boyhood on a farm on which the German-American tradition was to "work like hell and live by the tenets of Martin Luther."[34] The first part of that tradition and an aptitude for science carried him through Custer County High School, where he first encountered virology, and on to Montana State College (B.S. in Bacteriology and Chemistry, 1941).[35]

Graduating at the top of his class and armed with a national scholarship, Hilleman was admitted to the graduate program at the University of Chicago and awarded the additional financial assistance he badly needed. In those years – in the heyday of President Robert Maynard Hutchins – the university was elite, tough, and intensely individualistic. It was, in short, a setting well tailored for a talented,

---

33 Max Tishler, Oral History, July 13, 1988, MA; John T. Connor, Interview, Dec. 27, 1991. A. N. Richards to V. Bush, Aug. 14, 1955, Richards Papers, UPA.

34 The family had migrated from Hannover in the nineteenth century, settling first in southeast Missouri and moving to Montana before the First World War. M. R. Hilleman, "Notes," MA.

35 During his childhood, Hilleman was exposed to science by his older brothers, one of whom went on to become a professor of anatomy and physiology at Oregon State University. Farm life in Montana also involved an introduction to the mechanical arts through daily encounters with a blacksmithy and machine shop. Young Hilleman added to this practical knowledge an acquaintance with electricity by way of building radios and other electrical devices. Fascinated with science as a high school student, he read and reported on Wendell Stanley's first paper on crystallization of tobacco mosaic virus. At graduation, he received the award (Bausch & Lomb) given to the school's outstanding science major. Maurice R. Hilleman, Interview, Nov. 13 and 21, 1991; M. R. Hilleman, "Notes," MA.

hard-working farm boy who was dedicated to cutting-edge science. Ambitious and driven, Hilleman was determined to build a career that would take him far from the Big Sky country.

He would enter his new calling just as American science was beginning to experience a dramatic transformation. Wartime success with team research and large-scale federal funding had convinced leaders like Vannevar Bush – then director during the war of the federal government's Office of Scientific Research and Development - that in peacetime the nation's scientific establishment deserved similar support for similar types of focused research programs. In the years ahead, the government would provide extensive support for American science, and Hilleman and many others would ride that powerful wave of increased status and funding to the top of their professions.

At Chicago in the mid-1940s, however, Hilleman was just slightly ahead of this wave of scientific expansion. Personally, he was in a financial trough and with no family resources to fall back on, he found it necessary to work half time to sustain himself. He nevertheless completed a five-year program in three years, finishing his prize-winning dissertation on the psittacosis-lymphogranuloma venereum-trachoma group of agents in 1944.[36] In that final year as a student (Ph.D. in Bacteriology and Parasitology), he assisted his faculty director in teaching a graduate course in virology, a subdiscipline still so new that they could not find a suitable textbook.[37]

---

36 M. R. Hilleman and F. B. Gordon, "Immunologic Relations of the Psittacosis Lymphogranuloma Group of Viral Agents," *Proceedings of the Society for Experimental Biology and Medicine* 56 (1944): 159–61; M. R. Hilleman, "Immunological Studies on the Psittacosis-Lymphogranuloma Group of Viral Agents," *Journal of Infectious Diseases* 76, no. 2 (1945): 96–114. At Chicago, Hilleman discovered the immunological means to distinguish between the agents later known as chlamydiae. For this work the university awarded him the Howard Taylor Ricketts Prize.

37 According to M. R. Hilleman, "Notes," MA, the administration at Chicago first protested that he had not been in the program long enough to receive a doctorate but then awarded him his degree. Much later (1987) the university would give him a Distinguished Alumni Medal for lifetime achievement.

Hilleman then confounded the faculty at Chicago by rejecting academe and opting for a career in industry. His academic mentors tried to persuade him to seek a university position, but he was interested in the possibility of developing specific medical products and was not averse to earning some money – at last. He took a job with E. R. Squibb & Sons in New Brunswick, New Jersey, where he was a research associate with responsibilities in both viral research and product manufacture. At Squibb, he and a colleague brought out a centrifuged, purified influenza vaccine during the same period when Sharp & Dohme was pressing forward with its influenza vaccine for the military.[38] Hilleman also developed a Japanese B encephalitis vaccine for use by American troops in Asia and carried forward the basic research he had started at Chicago on chlamydiae.[39] In 1947 Squibb promoted him, making him chief of his operation. Now he was in charge of the company's smallpox and rabies vaccines, as well as quality control. While his experience with large-scale production and administration would later prove valuable, at this point Hilleman was not satisfied with the way his career was developing. He decided to return to basic research in a new setting.

In 1948, he moved to Walter Reed, at first to the Army Medical Service Graduate School (1948–55). There he launched a series of highly productive research programs on the adeno and influenza viruses. His output was impressive. At Walter Reed, he set the pace that would result over a long career in more than 450 scientific publications.[40] By

---

38 See the discussion of the use of the Sharples centrifuge to concentrate and purify the virus in U.S. Office of Scientific Research and Development, *Advances in Military Medicine*, 1:18–19.

39 On Japanese B type encephalitis see ibid., p. 34. M. R. Hilleman, "Notes," MA. See also Paul, *History of Poliomyelitis*, pp. 448–9. As Paul points out, the military later abandoned this research program to the dismay of Dr. Albert Sabin, who was then serving on the U.S. Army Epidemiological Board's Commission on Neurotropic Virus Diseases.

40 See M. R. Hilleman, "Curriculum Vitae," MA.

1956, when he became chief of Walter Reed's Department of Respiratory Diseases, he had a solidly established national and international reputation and was deeply engaged in the work of providing the central laboratory control for a worldwide influenza surveillance program.[41] Tishler was impressed with Hilleman's laboratory, his forceful manner, and his potential as a "mover."[42]

Well situated at Walter Reed, Hilleman mulled over Merck's offer for some time. The company had a strong tradition in research, dating back to the early 1930s. The firm's scientists had published extensively and many of their breakthrough drugs had been front-page news. But still Hilleman was cautious. His years at Squibb had certainly not been the most productive part of his life, and he was now in the prime of his scientific career. He was not going to allow anything to interfere with his progress in science. On this point, however, Tishler had a strong card to play. As president of MSDRL, he guaranteed that Hilleman would have "total freedom" to run both a basic and an applied vaccine research operation. He would not have to abandon science.[43] And along the way, he could do what would be best for his family.

---

41 Etheridge, *Sentinel for Health*, pp. 80–2.

42 Max Tishler, Oral History, July 13, 1988, MA. While Tishler was visiting Walter Reed to talk about the job, Hilleman received a phone call from an Army officer. Hilleman apparently told the Colonel: "Get off your butt and get out there and get some blood samples as quickly as possible. I need them. Don't give me any excuses." As Tishler later observed, "This impressed me a great deal."

43 See D. Hicks, "Published Papers, Tacit Competencies and Corporate Management of the Public/Private Character of Knowledge," *Industrial and Corporate Change* 4, no. 2 (1995): 401–24. Gambardella, *Science and Innovation*, pp. 83–8, comments on Merck's research organization in the 1980s, pointing out that the scientists had a relatively high degree of autonomy. As this episode with Hilleman and the subsequent development of Virus and Cell Biology Research indicate, the characteristics Gambardella identifies with the 1980s had deep roots in Merck's history.

This at last was an offer Hilleman could not refuse.[44] In 1957 he became director of Virus and Cell Biology Research in the Merck Institute for Therapeutic Research.[45] The Institute, a separate, subsidiary organization, had long been headed (1932–56) by Dr. Hans Molitor, a pharmacologist.[46] Even after the various laboratories at Merck and at Sharp & Dohme had been consolidated under MSDRL, the Institute had remained administratively and legally separate.[47] Now it would provide the center at West Point, Pennsylvania, for Hilleman's new program.

3

When Hilleman arrived at West Point, the company's pharmaceutical and biological division (Merck Sharp & Dohme, MSD) was deeply engaged in a new influenza vaccine project. Hilleman wasted no time getting up to speed on this project because he had actually discovered

---

44 As Hilleman recalls, he carefully pondered Tishler's offer, and while he thought about the situation, President Henry Gadsden of Merck kept increasing the proposed salary. Finally, the company reached a figure that Hilleman knew would provide a private-school education for his baby daughter, Jeryl Lynn, and he accepted. Maurice R. Hilleman, Interview, Nov. 13 and 21, 1991.

45 Maurice R. Hilleman, Interview, Nov. 13 and 21, 1991.

46 In 1956, Molitor became chairman of the Institute's board. For background on Molitor's appointment and tenure at Merck see Sturchio, ed., *Values and Visions*, pp. 23, 27, 67–8, 70, 74, and 81. H. Molitor, "On the Working Principles of the Merck Institute," Aug. 1, 1944; Dr. Hans Molitor, "Biographical Information," Aug. 24, 1960; in MA. A. N. Richards, "Remarks at the Groundbreaking of the New Merck Institute Laboratory at Rahway, Oct. 25, 1951"; A. N. Richards to H. Molitor, May 6, 1932; H. Molitor to A. N. Richards, July 12, 1932; in Richards Papers, UPA.

47 Under Molitor's direction, the Institute had over the years placed ever greater emphasis on fundamental, rather than applied, research. The West Point biological operation, on the other hand, had a distinctly applied orientation. With this in mind, management had following the 1953 merger decided to leave the two organizations geographically and administratively decentralized. Max Tishler, Oral History, July 13, 1988, MA.

the virus and played a large role in getting work started on a vaccine while he was still at Walter Reed. As Hilleman knew at that time, the country's Type A vaccines had been ineffective against an outbreak of flu in 1947 because of a shift in the chemical makeup of the antigen. The new viral subtype in 1947 – a result of antigenic shift – became known as influenza Type A_1.[48] Thus, in 1957, when a new influenza outbreak began in Hong Kong, he and his associates at Walter Reed had been prepared to deal with the problem of another shift. They had acted quickly. Hilleman requested throat specimens of the virus from the U.S. Army's 406th Medical General Laboratory in Zama, Japan. On May 13, 1957, his lab received the first specimen, and after nine fourteen-hour days, they had isolated and proved the existence of a new virus (Type A_2), labeled Asian influenza.[49]

Hilleman then made a decisive move: "I put out a press release to tell the world that there was going to be a pandemic when school started in the fall." That took nerve, but as he later observed: "I was young."[50] This virus, Hilleman and his team noted, had a radically different antigenic specificity. The changes since 1947 had been moderate drifts, but this was not the case in 1957. The evidence that they were dealing with a decisive shift was convincing – at least to the Walter Reed researchers. They conducted immunological cross-tests with chickens and ferrets, using prototype A virus strains; these tests indicated that the new strains were antigenically different. They also studied the sera from a diverse group of persons in the population and found a lack of antibody to the new virus. It had apparently not been previously encountered by the population. The evidence pointing to a profound shift was substantiated by the pandemic epidemiological

---

48 Hilleman, Mason, and Buescher, "Antigenic Pattern," pp. 829–35; Hilleman, "Pattern of Antigen Variation," pp. 798–803.

49 Etheridge, *Sentinel for Health*, pp. 80–1. At first Hilleman called it "Far East" influenza, then later changed the name. M. R. Hilleman, "Notes," MA.

50 Maurice R. Hilleman, Interview, Nov. 13 and 21, 1991.

spread of the virus.[51] Because the population lacked antibody to the virus, the disease resulted in severe illness and spread rapidly, with a high attack rate. They now concluded that immunity depended on exposure to the antigenic family, the type, and the subgroup of influenza.[52]

Given his laboratory's findings, Hilleman had quickly alerted the central institutions in the network dedicated to control of influenza. He notified the Armed Forces Epidemiological Board, the U.S. Public Health Service's Centers for Disease Control, the World Health Organization (WHO), and the six vaccine manufacturers – including Merck – of the existence of this new virus.[53] At that time, it was still impossible to predict accurately how severe the disease would be, but the experience of the 1918–19 pandemic was obviously in everyone's mind. Walter Reed provided strains of the new virus to the National Institutes of Health (NIH), which gave samples to Merck and the other manufacturers.[54] The Division of Biologics Standards (DBS, a division of NIH) asked Dr. Eugene S. Barclay, director of Merck Sharp & Dohme's Biological Production Division, if the company could produce a pilot batch of vaccine from the new strain.[55] Barclay and his

51 R. F. Betts and R. G. Douglas, "Influenza Virus," in Mandell, Douglas, and Bennett, eds., *Infectious Diseases*, p. 1309.

52 H. M. Meyer, Jr., M. R. Hilleman, M. L. Miesse, I. P. Crawford, and A. S. Bankhead, "New Antigenic Variant in Far East Influenza Epidemic, 1957," *Proceedings of the Society for Experimental Biology and Medicine* 95 (1957): 609–16.

53 The network quickly became more complex. The American Medical Association (AMA), the American Hospital Association (AHA), and the state health officers launched an educational campaign for all of the relevant personnel engaged in healthcare. Etheridge, *Sentinel for Health*, pp. 82–4.

54 M. R. Hilleman, F. J. Flatley, S. A. Anderson, M. L. Luecking, and D. J. Levinson, "Antibody Response in Volunteers to Asian Influenza Vaccine," *Journal of the American Medical Association* 166, no. 10 (1958): 1134–40.

55 As a result of the crisis over the Salk vaccine, the Biologics Control Laboratory had been reorganized; it became the Division of Biologics Standards in 1955. Smith, *Patenting the Sun*, p. 368.

colleagues said they were prepared to move ahead at once — at no cost to the government.[56]

Merck received the new virus strain on May 23, 1957. Two weeks later, on June 8, the company was able to deliver a batch of 2,500 shots of the experimental vaccine to the NIH (apparently this was the first order the government received). At this point, Merck's management decided to go ahead with production regardless of the government's decision and without a government subsidy.[57] This was a bold move involving considerable risk. If there was an epidemic, large quantities of vaccine would be needed. So Merck needed a large production program that would have to be initiated before it was certain that an epidemic would even occur in the United States. Getting into production quickly at this level would involve complex logistical problems. The firm would, for instance, be forced to hire a large number of new workers, a situation that was likely to create dissatisfaction among Merck's existing employees. But with influenza spreading swiftly through Japan, the Philippines, and much of the Orient, time was short. The company decided to launch its program at once.[58]

At Walter Reed, meanwhile, Hilleman and his colleagues were using the experimental vaccine to test for an antibody response with a group of volunteers. In addition to determining the efficacy of the new vaccine, the Walter Reed team sought to establish whether there was any benefit to be obtained from administering the old-formula polyvalent (A, A_1, and B) vaccine as a way of inducing antibodies

---

56 Harvard Business School, "Merck & Co., Inc." (Case Study, 1960); *Merck Review* 28, no. 1 (1968); both in MA. Maurice R. Hilleman, Interview, Nov. 13 and 21, 1991.

57 During the polio trials, the National Foundation had given the manufacturers a subsidy in the form of a guaranteed purchase contract, regardless of the outcome of the trials.

58 *Merck Review* 18, no. 4 (1957), MA. It was Hilleman's impression — confirmed by the output figures — that Merck Sharp & Dohme was more responsive than other firms in the industry to the call for a crash production program. M. R. Hilleman, "Notes," MA.

against the Asian virus or as a means of enhancing the antibody response to the new vaccine. Neither was found to be the case, but the new monovalent Asian influenza vaccine proved to be both effective and safe.[59]

As soon as NIH granted approval, Merck went into full-capacity production, launching a crash program of unprecedented scale. MSD's staff inoculated with the virus enormous numbers of embryonated, white-shelled hens' eggs that were eleven days old. The eggs were then incubated for two days, carefully inspected, and the infected allantoic fluid harvested.[60] The staff then killed the virus in the pooled material with formalin, precipitated it with protamine, and purified and tested the concentrate.[61] By this time the firm had acquired the new employees it needed and was purchasing 150,000 eggs a day – for a total of six million.

By the end of August 1957, Merck Sharp & Dohme was producing three million doses a week, but still there was a public uproar over the availability of vaccine in this country. The specter of 1918–19 generated controversy and widespread concern. The public was in "near hysteria" as to how and when the scarce vaccine would be distributed. The order of distribution, as determined by the network's dominant institutions, seems in retrospect to have been reasonable. The first Americans to receive the new product were members of the armed forces serving overseas in areas immediately threatened by the pandemic. After that, the military serving at home received shots, and then the vaccine was made available to the general public.

Reasonable as that might seem in retrospect, the furor prompted another powerful institution, the American Medical Association, to draft a new code to guide future distributions of scarce vaccines.

---

59 Hilleman, Flatley, Anderson, Leucking, and Levinson, "Antibody Response," pp. 1134–40. See also Etheridge, *Sentinel for Health*, p. 84.

60 The eggs were inspected for retained viability.

61 *Merck Review* 18, no. 4 (1957); Harvard Business School, "Merck & Co., Inc."; in MA.

There was nothing to criticize in Merck's performance during 1957. Indeed, by the end of the year, the firm had released more than twenty million doses — nearly half that supplied by the entire industry.[62] But the intense public concern, the involvement of the leading association of physicians (Merck's primary market), and the complex interactions that had characterized this particular network of institutions made it clear that a scientist/spokesperson of Hilleman's stature would be needed if the company's program in virus and cell biology was going to be successful in the years ahead.

Leadership of the kind that Merck needed could not be provided by scientists of lesser stature and energy — no matter how many of them the firm might hire. Innovation along these particular lines required a special type of leadership. The company could subdivide along functional lines its activities in science, science management, and science diplomacy or representation. But it needed one forceful leader. Without firm direction, good scientific decisions, and effective representation inside and outside the firm, Virus and Cell Biology at Merck was likely in the years ahead to remain what it had been since 1953 — a minor element in the organization's competitive strategy.

Historians have of late paid far too little attention to this type of leadership. The popularity of social history "from the bottom up," the interest in culture and diversity, the reaction against history as a study of the accomplishments of great white men, and the enthusiasm in some quarters for impersonal, behavioral explanations of organizational performance have all undercut scholarly analysis of the decisive role of leadership in modern institutions. This is particularly true where large-scale organizations — public and private — are concerned. The organizations and their leaders have contributed to this tendency,

---

62 World Health Organization, Expert Committee on Respiratory Virus Diseases, "First Report," *World Health Organization Technical Report Series* 170 (1959). Etheridge, *Sentinel for Health*, pp. 84–6, describes the public tension that developed over the distribution of the new vaccine. Meanwhile, the experience in 1957–8 appears to have strengthened public support for institutions like the CDC.

---

masking their behavior behind public relations baffles and avoiding the conspicuous personal activities that once characterized the country's elites.

But viewed from the inside out, organizations like Merck & Co., Inc., are a complex, shifting combination of divisions and departments, each of which needs effective leadership if it is to contribute to the firm's ability to promote and sustain innovative behavior. One of the most important functions of the firm's CEO and top executives is to select leaders like Hilleman, to provide them with the support they need, and then to step aside and let them develop the firm's new capabilities. That is what Merck's CEO, John Connor, its president, Henry Gadsden, and the head of the laboratories, Max Tishler, did in 1957. They would have good reason to be satisfied with their decision, but the payoff on this new venture would not begin for several years.

HILLEMAN'S INNOVATIONS: FIRST PHASE

AX TISHLER and Merck's top executives were certain that they had found the right man to rev up the company's research in virology. But Maurice Hilleman's first venture at West Point was a failure – at least from the company's perspective. When the new director of Virus and Cell Biology Research arrived at the firm's laboratories, he discovered that Betty Hampil and two of her colleagues were continuing to work on the Salk polio vaccine.[1] The vaccine was still unpredictable and its potency too variable. They were attempting to purify the virus, to use precise, standardized amounts of each serotype, and thus to obtain a vaccine of "uniform high potency."[2]

While one member of the research team, Jesse Charney, had discovered a novel way of precipitating the polio virus, the project was

---

1 Hampil was working with Dr. Alfred A. Tytell and Jesse Charney.

2 M. R. Hilleman, J. Charney, A. A. Tytell, C. Weihl, D. Cornfeld, J. T. Ichter, H. D. Riley, Jr., and N. Huang, "Investigation into the Development and Clinical Testing of a Poliomyelitis Vaccine Containing Standardized Amounts of Purified Poliomyelitis Virus Antigens," *Academy of Medicine of New Jersey Bulletin* 6, no. 3 (1960): 107–8. There had been cases of paralytic polio among persons who had received doses of the Salk vaccine, and the problem had been traced to the lack of uniformity. See also M. R. Hilleman to M. Tishler, Sept. 22, 1958, MA.

not moving ahead in a manner satisfactory to Hilleman.[3] As he pushed forward with his efforts to reorganize and accelerate the work in virology, he took over direction of the Salk vaccine program. As that research progressed, Merck decided to concentrate its resources on this single program, leaving the production of oral Sabin vaccine to its competitors.[4] After three years of additional research and clinical trials, Hilleman's team had a purified Salk vaccine that proved safe and effective in the clinical tests. The U.S. Public Health Service released Merck's new product for use by doctors in 1960.[5]

But just as *Purivax* was nearing release, Hilleman and his coworkers made a startling discovery. They found evidence of a wild indigenous virus in the monkey kidney cells used to grow polio virus. The newly discovered virus, later identified as SV_{40}, seemed at first to present no serious problem for *Purivax* or the other polio vaccines. There was no evidence that SV_{40} had caused any problems in the millions of persons who had been given either the Salk or Sabin vaccines to date. This included those being immunized in the huge Soviet

---

3 J. Charney, A. A. Tytell, R. A. Machlowitz, and M. R. Hilleman, "Development of a Purified Poliomyelitis Virus Vaccine," *Journal of the American Medical Association* 177, no. 9 (1961): 592.

4 J. T. Connor to Surgeon General Leroy E. Burney, Nov. 25, 1959, MA. As Connor pointed out, Merck had produced oral polio vaccine for the field studies in the United States and had provided financial support for Sabin's studies in Mexico. But Pfizer, Pitman-Moore, Lederle, and Wyeth now appeared to be ready to produce the live vaccine in sufficient quantities to meet the nation's needs.

5 See also M. Tishler to M. R. Hilleman, Dec. 30, 1959, MA. M. R. Hilleman to M. Tishler, July 18, 1960, MA. Hilleman, Charney, Tytell, Weihl, Cornfeld, Ichter, Riley, and Huang, "Investigation into the Development," pp. 106–36. Charney, Tytell, Machlowitz, and Hilleman, "Development of a Purified," pp. 591–5. M. R. Hilleman, J. Charney, A. A. Tytell, C. Weihl, D. Cornfeld, J. T. Ichter, H. D. Riley, Jr., N. Huang, H. Cramblett, and H. Moffet, "Purified Poliomyelitis Vaccine" (paper presented to the American Public Health Association, Nov. 1, 1960); and Merck, Sharp & Dohme, "Press Release," July 13, 1960; both in MA.

campaign then underway. Moreover, it was not evident whether or not the SV_{40} was inactivated in the process of making *Purivax*.[6]

Merck nevertheless went into a damage-control mode. The company sent Hilleman to alert responsible officials in the virology network and to coordinate a response. Two days after finding evidence of SV_{40}, Hilleman was at NIH to discuss the problem with, among others, his former mentor at Walter Reed, Joseph Smadel. The consensus was that "we had an observed phenomenon, the interpretation of which was in doubt and the significance of which was unknown." What then to do? They "had to weigh the factual damage of removing the means to prevent polio this coming season against the theoretical problem of continuing injection of vaccine suspected of containing live SV_{40}." There was agreement that if Merck removed its vaccine from the market unilaterally, all of the other producers of Salk vaccine would have to follow suit. Instead, they decided to conduct the further tests that might lead to "a definitive judgment."[7] In the meantime, Merck stopped sending Salk vaccine to its distribution centers and quietly quarantined shipments from any of those plants. While awaiting the next round of tests, the company decided not to withdraw the supplies in the hands of hospitals, doctors, and pharmacies.[8]

------

6 M. R. Hilleman to M. Tishler, June 19, 1961, MA. M. R. Hilleman, "Professor Chumakov, Live Poliomyelitis Vaccine, and the Problem of Indigenous Monkey Viruses" (draft of paper presented to the Chumakov Memorial Conference, Institute of Poliomyelitis and Viral Encephalitides [Moscow], Nov. 15–17, 1994).

7 M. R. Hilleman to M. Tishler, May 22, 1961; and M. Tishler to H. W. Gadsden, May 22, 1961; both in MA. At this point in the discussions, NIH, the head of its Division of Biological Standards (DBS), Dr. R. Murray, and the NIH Technical Committee had concluded that there was no evidence that the virus caused any disease in humans.

8 M. Tishler to H. W. Gadsden, June 23, 1961; J. J. Horan, Memorandum for files, June 26, 1961; C. S. Keefer to Board of Directors, June 26, 1961. See also J. A. Shannon, Chairman, "Report of the Technical Committee on Poliomyelitis Vaccine," May 18, 1961; and Director, DBS, to Manufacturers of Poliomyelitis and Adenovirus Vaccine, May 20, 1961. All in MA.

The additional tests converted a problem into a crisis. It was a crisis for Merck and for the entire network of institutions involved in polio vaccination in the United States and abroad. By this time, the concerned parties in the United States included the head of NIH, the Surgeon General of the United States, Senator Hill, the Secretary of Health, Education, and Welfare, various public health officials, and of course all of the clinical investigators using Merck's vaccine.[9] Hilleman's additional research and similar work conducted at NIH now indicated that SV_{40} induced tumors of varying degrees of malignancy in hamsters.[10]

This raised the possibility that a cancer-producing substance had been given to millions of persons and would be given to more in the United States, in the USSR, and elsewhere in the months ahead.[11] Although Hilleman was convinced that the problem of SV_{40} could be solved, the company could no longer tolerate the risk. After several

---

9 M. R. Hilleman, Memorandum for file, June 27, 1961; K. H. Beyer to M. Tishler, June 30, 1961. The situation was also being discussed in the popular and medical press; see chronology, June 30, 1961. All in MA.

10 B. H. Sweet and M. R. Hilleman, "Detection of a 'Non-Detectable' Simian Virus (Vacuolating Agent) Present in Rhesus and Cynomolgus Monkey-Kidney Cell Culture Material: A Preliminary Report," *Second International Conference on Live Poliovirus Vaccines*, Pan American Health Organization and the World Health Organization, Washington, DC, June 6–7, 1960, pp. 79–85; B. H. Sweet and M. R. Hilleman, "The Vacuolating Virus, SV_{40}," *Proceedings of the Society for Experimental Biology and Medicine* 105 (1960): 420–7. A. J. Girardi, M. R. Hilleman, and R. E. Zwickey, "Tests in Hamsters for Oncogenic Quality of Ordinary Viruses Including Adenovirus Type 7," *Proceedings of the Society for Experimental Biology and Medicine* 115 (1964): 1141–50.

11 M. R. Hilleman, Memorandum for file, June 13, 1961; and A. J. Girardi, B. H. Sweet, V. B. Slotnick, and M. R. Hilleman, "Development of Tumors in Hamsters Inoculated in the Neonatal Period with Vacuolating Virus, SV_{40}" (draft of paper for the *Proceedings of the Society for Experimental Biology and Medicine*); both in MA. See also *Lancet* (Apr. 7, 1962): 730–1. S. L. Katz, "Efficacy, Potential and Hazards of Vaccines," *New England Journal of Medicine* 270, no. 17 (1964): 884–9.

agonizing discussions, the firm removed *Purivax* from the market and abandoned polio vaccine entirely.[12]

Defeated in his first commercial venture at Merck, Hilleman could later take some solace in the scientific developments that would flow from the discovery of SV_{40}. This simian virus would become an important element in research on viral causes of cancer and would be used extensively in studies of the molecular biology and genetics of DNA viruses. Many years later, that line of research would resurface at Merck in the form of promising oncology studies.[13] But in 1961, the West Point laboratory could squeeze little happiness from reflections on good science. Virus and Cell Biology Research at Merck had struck out in its first time at bat.

1

Fortunately for Hilleman and his research team, the game was far from over. In addition to the research on polio vaccine, Hilleman had

---

12 In 1962, Hilleman's position on SV_{40} would be supported by the NIH Task Force on Tissue Culture Viruses and Vaccines. See "Continuously Cultured Tissue Cells and Viral Vaccines," *Science* 139 (Jan. 4, 1963): 15–20. See also J. F. Fraumeni, Jr., F. Ederer, and R. Miller, "An Evaluation of the Carcinogenicity of Simian Virus 40 in Man," *JAMA* 185, no. 9 (1963): 713–18. Also "Polio Vaccine, SV 40, Cancer: A Report," *JAMA* 196, no. 2 (1966): 37.

Years later, Jonas Salk would try to persuade the firm to go back into production of his killed-virus vaccine. His contention at the time was that the Salk product was safer than the Sabin oral polio vaccine, which had become virtually the only one used in the United States. Merck decided, however, not to reenter this field. See M. R. Hilleman to Those Concerned, Apr. 24 and May 8, 1975; J. E. Lyons to J. Salk, May 30, 1975; all in MA. See also *Science* 196 (Apr. 1, 1977): 35–6.

13 A similar delayed sequence took place in the biochemistry of cholesterol synthesis. In 1956, scientists at MSDRL discovered mevalonic acid, a crucial intermediate in cholesterol biosynthesis. Later, it would be discovered that mevalonic acid is formed by the enzyme HMG-CoA reductase, and much later (1978–9), A. W. Alberts and his colleagues at Merck would discover lovastatin, an HMG-CoA reductase inhibitor. In 1987, *Mevacor* (lovastatin) would be the first such inhibitor to receive FDA approval.

been busy transforming what he perceived as a "piddling operation" into a first-rate virology department. This involved some dramatic changes in the staff.[14] It was also necessary to sharpen the organization's focus. When Hilleman arrived, he found that the virologists were doing a considerable amount of "chemotherapy work," searching for chemicals that would demonstrate antiviral activity. That was consistent with Merck's background in research and with the talents of the president of MSDRL, Max Tishler. At first, Hilleman tried to upgrade that part of his program, but he recognized that it was a "futile effort" at a time when they could not distinguish cellular from viral metabolism. Viruses are genetic entities and Hilleman decided he would get enthusiastic about antiviral screening when someone was able to "cure brown eyes."[15] By phasing out this part of the operation, he was able to concentrate more resources on the programs he thought had some likelihood of success in the near future.[16]

For those programs, it was necessary to improve the firm's clinical research and its ties to the pediatrics network. In order to do so

14 Maurice R. Hilleman, Interview, Nov. 13 and 21, 1991, discusses the changes in the staff.

15 M. R. Hilleman, Interview, Nov. 13 and 21, 1991; and M. R. Hilleman, "Notes," MA. For a more optimistic, contemporary view of the potential of viral chemotherapy see I. Tamm and H. J. Eggers, "Specific Inhibition of Replication of Animal Viruses," *Science* 142 (Oct. 4, 1963): 24–33; and 145 (Sept. 25, 1964): 1443–4.

16 It was essential to the firm's future success that the leaders of the previous or overlapping cycle of innovation did not impose their own priorities on the leader who was attempting to develop new capabilities for the organization. Tishler was a strong president of MSDRL and he was tempted in this instance to carry forward his style of research and science. But he wisely backed off and gave Hilleman the support and autonomy he needed. In regard to autonomy see Gambardella, *Science and Innovation*, pp. 83–8.

Later, when the biochemistry of the cell was better understood, there would be important developments in antiviral drugs. On the problems with viral chemotherapy see Alfred Grafe, *A History of Experimental Virology* (New York, 1991), pp. 277–85.

as quickly as possible, Hilleman separated vaccine clinical operations from the existing clinical organization in Merck Sharp & Dohme.[17] He had his sights on some of the leading diseases of children, infections that usually found their way to the pediatricians' doors, and he wanted first-class clinical support from researchers with strong credentials among pediatricians. He launched this effort while working on the polio problem by establishing contact with an old friend from his Walter Reed days. Dr. Joseph Stokes, now physician-in-chief of the Children's Hospital and chairman of the Department of Pediatrics of the University of Pennsylvania School of Medicine, had directed the Hepatitis Commission when Hilleman was in Washington, D.C.[18] They decided to form a joint clinical team to work on the number one communicable disease killer and crippler of children.

Deaths from the complications of measles far exceeded those from poliomyelitis.[19] In the early 1960s, it was calculated that the disease had or would attack approximately 95 percent of the U.S. population, with an annual average of four million cases.[20] While for many children measles was uncomfortable and temporary, for others

17 This decision also indicated that Hilleman had more leeway than he would have had in many firms. Gambardella, *Science and Innovation*, pp. 83–8.

18 See A. M. Bongiovanni, "Joseph Stokes, Jr.," *Pediatrics* 50, no. 1 (1972): 163–4, an obituary letter. Stokes had in 1939 started the first diagnostic virus laboratory in a clinical department in the United States. He had worked on measles for some years prior to his arrangement with Merck; see E. P. Maris, S. S. Gellis, F. Shaffer, W. B. Dunham, J. Stokes, Jr., and G. Rake, "Vaccination of Children with Various Chorioallantoic Passages of Measles Virus," *Pediatrics* 4, no. 1 (1949): 1–8.

19 F. C. Robbins, "Viruses of the Acute Communicable Diseases," *Pediatrics* 25, no. 1 (1960): 119–26. R. J. Warren and F. C. Robbins, "Prevention of Viral Diseases," *Pediatrics* 30, no. 6 (1962): 862–74. J. Stokes, Jr., R. Weibel, R. Halenda, C. M. Reilly, and M. R. Hilleman, "Studies of Live Attenuated Measles Virus Vaccine in Man: 1. Clinical Aspects," *American Journal of Public Health* 52, no. 2 (1962): 29–43.

20 "For Your Information," 1963, p. 4, MA.

the virus's effects were devastating and permanent. In the United States and abroad, measles was responsible for up to 50 percent of childhood morbidity and mortality from this type of illness. Sometimes the virus caused fatal pneumonia. Sometimes it undermined immunological systems, laying the way for secondary bacterial infections. Other effects included encephalitis – inflammation of the brain, which can have a wide range of consequences, from temporary problems to death – and otitis media – inflammation of the middle ear, which can result in violent earache and in permanent deafness.[21]

While measles had been described for many hundreds of years, it had until the twentieth century been viewed almost universally as an inevitable disease.[22] In the early 1900s, serum prophylaxis had occasionally been tried in Europe, and the H. K. Mulford Company had experimented with a measles serum in the late 1920s.[23] But even today there is no known treatment available.[24] Some of the first systematic efforts in the U.S. to protect against measles issued from the military. During World War II, the Armed Forces laboratories tried to develop an egg-passaged, attenuated live-virus vaccine, and Drs. Joseph Stokes and John F. Enders obtained from fractionated plasma a preparation of

---

21 A. A. Gershon, "Measles Virus (Rubeola)," in Mandell, Douglas, and Bennett, eds., *Infectious Diseases*, pp. 1279–82.

22 Measles had often been conflated or confused with smallpox and scarlet fever.

23 See J. Reichel (Mulford) to G. W. McCoy (Director, the Hygienic Laboratory), Feb. 26 and Mar. 21, 1927; Major H. C. Michie to Drs. Degkwitz and Harrison, n.d.; H. C. Michie to G. W. McCoy, Mar. 26, 1927; G. W. McCoy to Lieutenant Colonel J. F. Siler, Mar. 25, 1927; G. W. McCoy to J. Reichel, Mar. 25, 1927; excerpt from Mulford advertising for Anti-Measles Serum (Degkwitz). The serum, which was obtained from sheep, was being made under license from Dr. Rudolf Degkwitz of Greifswald, Germany. All in RG 443 (Records of the NIH, 1930–48), National Archives. This particular serum does not appear in H. K. Mulford, Price-List, 1929, MA. See also G. Edsall, "Passive Immunization," *Pediatrics* 32, no. 4 (1963): 603.

24 Gershon, "Measles Virus (Rubeola)," p. 1284; Parish, *Victory with Vaccines*, pp. 184–6.

measles antibodies that could provide a degree of passive immunity and some modification of the disease. The vaccine was, however, too reactogenic and the globulin treatment was expensive and unreliable.[25]

Following the war, John Enders continued his work on viruses and from his laboratory in Boston came the breakthrough in tissue culture techniques that transformed the search for new vaccines.[26] His research team was now able to propagate and pass through successive cell cultures the viruses with which they were working. After their Nobel prize-winning innovations with polio virus, Enders and his colleagues turned their attention to measles. Using throat washings and blood samples from David Edmonston, a Boston-area schoolboy with measles, Enders, Samuel Katz, Thomas Peebles, and their associates were able to isolate the virus, the necessary preliminary step to growing pure cultures.

Then they cultivated the virus and began the process of attenuating it. In Enders's laboratory at the Children's Hospital, they seeded the Edmonston measles virus into successive human kidney cultures, then into serial cultures of the human amnion, and finally adapted it to chick-embryo cell cultures.[27] The goal — to attenuate the virus to the point that it would prompt antibody production without causing the disease — took some time to achieve. Milan Milanovic spent three years passaging the virus through a variety of different tissue types. Finally, in 1958, the tests indicated that their live-virus vaccine would be successful in neutralizing the measles virus.

---

25 U.S. Office of Scientific Research and Development, *Advances in Military Medicine*, 1:412–16. Edsall, "Passive Immunization," p. 603.

26 M. R. Hilleman, J. Stokes, Jr., E. B. Buynak, R. Weibel, R. Halenda, and H. Goldner, "Studies of Live Attenuated Measles Virus Vaccine in Man: 2. Appraisal of Efficacy," *American Journal of Public Health* 52, no. 2 (1962): 44–56.

27 J. F. Enders and T. C. Peebles, "Propagation in Tissue Cultures of Cytopathogenic Agents from Patients with Measles," *Proceedings of the Society for Experimental Biology and Medicine* 86 (1954): 277–86. M. R. Hilleman, Interview, Nov. 13 and 21, 1991.

Pediatrician Saul Krugman, who worked closely with Enders, and M. T. Hoekenga guided the vaccine through its initial clinical tests. The vaccine successfully elicited neutralizing antibodies, but as the clinicians discovered, some of the recipients had a severe reaction, including fevers as high as 106° F.[28] Physicians as well as parents found the fevers and rashes unacceptable.[29] Moreover, there was still some question as to whether the vaccine produced thus far in laboratory conditions could be made on a scale that would yield sufficient supplies for large populations.

This was where Merck Sharp & Dohme's facilities and expertise came into play. Drs. Frankel and Hampil at MSD had been working as early as 1957 on the problems of propagating the measles virus in order to develop a practical killed-virus vaccine. Following Enders's techniques, they adapted his Edmonston virus to chick-embryo cells and conducted extensive tests for purity.[30] Hilleman, seldom a pessimist, was "very dubious" about the chances of success for any killed-measles vaccine, and in this case his suspicions were

28 J. F. Enders, S. L. Katz, M. V. Milovanovic, and A. Holloway, "Studies on an Attenuated Measles-Virus Vaccine," *New England Journal of Medicine* 263, no. 4 (1960): 153–9; pp. 159–84 in the same issue report on the clinical studies. M. R. Hilleman to M. Tishler, May 28, 1959, MA. See also the editorials in *JAMA* 174, no. 15 (1960): 136–7; and 177, no. 8 (1961): 569–70. And *Lancet* (Aug. 13, 1960): 354–5.

29 Hilleman, Stokes, Buynak, Weibel, Halenda, and Goldner, "Studies of Live Attenuated Measles Virus Vaccine in Man: 2. Appraisal of Efficacy," pp. 44–56. "Testing a Measles Vaccine," *Lancet* (Aug. 13, 1960): 354–5. Robbins, "Viruses of the Acute Communicable Diseases," pp. 119–26. A. J. F. Schwarz, P. A. Boyer, L. W. Zirbel, and C. J. York, "Experimental Vaccination Against Measles," *JAMA* 173, no. 8 (1960): 81–7; pp. 88–92 in the same issue report on a trial in Panama. Chase, *Magic Shots*, p. 312.

30 "Report to the Scientific Advisors of the Merck Institute," June 10, 1957, UPA. M. R. Hilleman to M. Tishler, Apr. 10, Sept. 22, and Dec. 31, 1958; all in MA.

correct. When tested, the Merck vaccine showed no evidence of protective efficacy.[31]

Meanwhile, Hilleman had guided his reorganized Virus and Cell Biology teams into an effort to produce a live-virus vaccine. Using Enders's original Edmonston B virus, they passed the virus twenty-four times in primary human kidney cells in culture, twenty-eight times in human amnion cell culture, twelve times in embryonated hens' eggs, and seventeen times in chick embryo. Having mastered the technologies of virus propagation and quantitative virus assay, they stabilized and lyophilized their vaccine and subjected it to safety testing. The result was a dried live-virus vaccine ready for clinical trials.

Joseph Stokes, Robert Weibel, and their associates at the Children's Hospital of Philadelphia were prepared to cooperate in testing the vaccine. They worked closely with the new outfit that MSD had organized within Virus and Cell Biology to handle protocols and analysis of the data. In the initial studies, carried out with small numbers of infants, they attempted to relate age to the level of maternally acquired measles immunity and to determine whether the presence of maternal antibody would allow active immunization to take place. Clearly, maternal antibody prevented a vaccine take. But the seroepidemiologic

31 M. R. Hilleman, J. Stokes, Jr., E. B. Buynak, C. M. Reilly, and B. Hampil, "Immunogenic Response to Killed Measles-Virus Vaccine," *American Journal of Diseases of Children* 103 (Mar. 1962): 444–51. M. R. Hilleman, "Notes," and M. R. Hilleman to M. Tishler, Apr. 25, 1958, with enclosure; both in MA. See also V. A. Fulginiti, J. J. Eller, A. W. Downie, and C. H. Kempe, "Altered Reactivity to Measles Virus," *JAMA* 202, no. 12 (1967): 101–6; and the editorial on p. 124 in the same issue.

But for a different indication see "Measles Vaccines," *Lancet* (Apr. 7, 1962): 730–1; W. Winkelstein, Jr., D. T. Karzon, D. Rush, and W. E. Mosher, "A Field Trial of Inactivated Measles Virus Vaccine in Young School Children," *JAMA* 194, no. 5 (1965): 494–8; and R. G. Lennon, P. Isacson, T. Rosales, W. R. Elsea, D. T. Karzon, and W. Winkelstein, Jr., "Skin Tests with Measles and Poliomyelitis Vaccines in Recipients of Inactivated Measles Virus Vaccine," *JAMA* 200, no. 4 (1967): 99–104.

studies showed that after nine months of age these antibodies were lost and the vaccine could be effective.[32] The clinical studies also showed, however, that the reactions (rashes, fevers, and rare febrile convulsions) were excessive.[33] MSD now had a vaccine that unfortunately resembled Sharp & Dohme's wartime flu vaccine. Both could prevent the disease but would not be widely used because of their reactogenicity.

At this crucial point in the process of innovation, the value of MSD's recently established links to a talented clinical team stood out clearly. Stokes was able to call upon his own wartime experience with immune globulin to suggest an answer to the problems with the new vaccine. The solution was to inject human immune gamma globulin into one arm and then immediately to inject the vaccine into the other. The gamma globulin attenuated the vaccine-induced measles without impairing the active immune response.

With the problem of reactogenicity apparently solved, the clinicians moved on to a larger, controlled field trial to determine protective efficacy. Merck's head of Virus and Cell Biology was a hands-on scientist, and when he learned that nearby Haverford Township kept records on measles occurrence, he headed for the township office. There he analyzed the measles history in the community. Knowing the size of the population, the birth rate, and the past occurrence of

---

32 The entire Merck program is reviewed and analyzed in M. R. Hilleman to M. Tishler, May 11, 1960, MA. J. Stokes, Jr., C. M. Reilly, M. R. Hilleman, and E. B. Buynak, "Use of Living Attenuated Measles-Virus Vaccine in Early Infancy," New England Journal of Medicine 263, no. 5 (1960): 230–3; C. M. Reilly, J. Stokes, Jr., E. B. Buynak, H. Goldner, and M. R. Hilleman, "Living Attenuated Measles-Virus Vaccine in Early Infancy: Studies of the Role of Passive Antibody in Immunization," New England Journal of Medicine 265, no. 4 (1961): 165–9. "Measles Immunization," Lancet (Dec. 2, 1961): 1246–7.

33 Stokes, Reilly, Hilleman, and Buynak, "Use of Living Attenuated Measles-Virus Vaccine in Early Infancy," pp. 230–3; Reilly, Stokes, Buynak, Goldner, and Hilleman, "Living Attenuated Measles-Virus in Early Infancy," pp. 165–9; J. Stokes, Jr., C. M. Reilly, E. B. Buynak, and M. R. Hilleman, "Immunologic Studies of Measles," American Journal of Hygiene 74, no. 3 (1961): 293–303. See also M. R. Hilleman to M. Tishler, Sept. 21, 1960, MA.

---

measles, he put together estimates of the percentage of susceptibles by age in the community and the likely attack rates of measles in the next winter period. With that figure in hand for expected cases per 300, he planned a placebo-controlled study using 600 children. Half of the children in the study were given the Frankel-Hampil killed-virus vaccine that had no potency and thus served as the placebo control. The results were excellent: the projections were almost on the nose and there was overwhelming proof of efficacy.[34]

The clinical studies also demonstrated that the combination of vaccine and gamma globulin was extremely effective.[35] Protection was

---

34 The dangers, liability problems, and difficulties of regulation in vaccine development were illustrated at this time by the efforts of another company to introduce an improved killed-virus measles vaccine. The product was potent; it induced neutralizing antibodies against the surface hemagglutinins; it thus provided protection and the government licensed it for general use. But nearly a year later, researchers discovered that children who had received the vaccine developed a serious *atypical* measles on exposure to natural measles or on revaccination with live vaccine. The Division of Biologics Standards immediately removed the product from the market, but the problem provided an apt illustration of the difficulties of controlling innovation in a network focused on an area of medical science still in an early stage of development.

Long-term measles immunity depends mostly on antibody directed against the fusion antigen; antibody against hemagglutinin is only of short duration. The formaldehyde used to kill the virus in the vaccine destroyed the fusion antigen and set the patient up for the often severe measles that occurred a year or so later. M. R. Hilleman, "Notes," MA. See also Hilleman, Stokes, Buynak, Reilly, and Hampil, "Immunogenic Response to Killed Measles-Virus Vaccine," pp. 444–51; and Gershon, "Measles Virus (Rubeola)," p. 1282.

35 On the use of gamma globulin at Merck and elsewhere see M. R. Hilleman to M. Tishler, et al., Oct. 17 and Nov. 2, 1960; both in MA. J. Stokes, Jr., M. R. Hilleman, R. E. Weibel, E. B. Buynak, R. Halenda, and H. Goldner, "Efficacy of Live, Attenuated Measles-Virus Vaccine Given with Human Immune Globulin: A Preliminary Report," *New England Journal of Medicine* 265, no. 11 (1961): 507–13. P. B. Kamin, B. T. Fein, and H. A. Britton, "Live, Attenuated Measles Vaccine," *JAMA* 185, no. 8 (1963): 99–102. See also: *Lancet* (Dec. 2, 1961): 1246–7; Warren and Robbins, "Prevention of Viral Diseases," pp. 868–70. And S. Krugman, J. P. Giles, A. M. Jacobs, and H. Friedman, "Studies with

not conferred if the globulin and vaccine were injected in the same syringe.[36] But when the shots were given concurrently and separately, the clinical reactions were insignificant – a mild, temporary fever or rash.[37] The follow-up studies on the children who had received the attenuated-virus vaccine were equally encouraging: one year and then two years later, these subjects had retained their immunity.[38]

When the initial tests were completed, MSD and the clinicians began the fine tuning that goes into preparing a vaccine for general release. In 1961, for instance, they still had not determined an appropriate, standardized ratio between the amount of gamma globulin and the amount of virus in the vaccine.[39] Nor did they have in place the

---

a Further Attenuated Live Measles-Virus Vaccine," *Pediatrics* 31, no. 6 (1963): 919–28; and Press release from the Children's Hospital of Philadelphia, Sept. 14, 1961, MA. See also M. R. Hilleman to M. Tishler, et al., Mar. 17, Oct. 4, Nov. 7 and 17, 1960, MA, on Saul Krugman's Nigerian trials.

36 Hilleman, Stokes, Buynak, Weibel, Halenda, and Goldner, "Studies of Live Attenuated Measles Virus Vaccine in Man: 2. Appraisal of Efficacy," pp. 44–56.

37 Stokes, Weibel, Halenda, Reilly, and Hilleman, "Studies of Live Attenuated Measles Virus Vaccine in Man: 1. Clinical Aspects," pp. 29–43; J. Stokes, Jr., R. Weibel, R. Halenda, C. M. Reilly, and M. R. Hilleman, "Enders' Live Measles-Virus Vaccine with Human Immune Globulin: I. Clinical Reactions," *American Journal of Diseases of Children* 103 (Mar. 1962): 366–72; Hilleman, Stokes, Buynak, Reilly, and Hampil, "Immunogenic Response to Killed Measles-Virus Vaccine," pp. 444–51.

38 J. Stokes, Jr., M. R. Hilleman, R. E. Weibel, E. B. Buynak, and R. Halenda, "Persistent Immunity Following Enders' Live, Attenuated Measles-Virus Vaccine Given with Human Immune Globulin," *New England Journal of Medicine* 267, no. 5 (1962): 222–4; R. E. Weibel, J. Stokes, Jr., R. Halenda, E. B. Buynak, and M. R. Hilleman, "Durable Immunity Two Years After Administration of Enders' Live Measles-Virus Vaccine with Immune Globulin," *New England Journal of Medicine* 270, no. 4 (1964): 172–5. See also J. S. Marks, T. J. Halpin, and W. A. Orenstein, "Measles Vaccine Efficacy in Children Previously Vaccinated at 12 Months of Age," *Pediatrics* 62, no. 6 (1978): 955–60.

39 M. R. Hilleman to M. Tishler and K. Beyer, Dec. 22, 1960, MA. The gamma globulin in the study contained 4,000 units of measles neutralizing

controls needed to ensure that the final product would be safe. At this point, even the government was not prepared to provide standards for controlling the vaccine's manufacture.

With success in sight, the firm quickly launched an intensive program to develop the necessary control procedures for production of a potent, safe vaccine. One of the fundamental safety controls involved the differentiation between and identification of virulent and attenuated measles virus strains. Researchers from three separate Merck organizations – something of an internal network – collaborated on this program.[40] The Division of Virus and Tissue Culture Research in the Merck Institute worked closely with MSDRL's Division of Toxicology and Pathology and with MSD's Veterinary Department in a successful effort to solve this problem.[41] The Veterinary Department's studies in vitro were useful to the research team when it presented its accumulated findings to the DBS, which was establishing regulatory criteria for the new product. Two other questions that had to be resolved before the dried vaccine could be released for public use involved how long and under what conditions it would remain properly infective. These studies indicated that the vaccine remained stable in storage for at least

---

antibody per ml. The volume dosage used to modify the vaccine response was 0.02 ml or 80 units per pound of the child's weight.

40 It is customary for scholars to treat large business organizations as if they are single entities, completely coordinated and controlled from above. Those who work in the organizations realize that they are in fact collections of sometimes competing and sometimes cooperating divisions, departments, and units. All have their own objectives and agendas. Principal-agent problems exist for these various subdivisions of corporations, just as they do for the individuals who work for them. L. Galambos, "The Authority and Responsibility of the Chief Executive Officer: Shifting Patterns in Large U.S. Enterprises in the Twentieth Century," *Industrial and Corporate Change* 4, no. 1 (1995): 190–1.

41 E. B. Buynak, H. M. Peck, A. A. Creamer, H. Goldner, and M. R. Hilleman, "Differentiation of Virulent from Avirulent Measles Strains," *American Journal of Diseases of Children* 103 (1962): 460–72.

---

eleven months at $4°$ C.[42] While this might present problems in under-developed parts of the world, there would be no difficulty in ensuring proper storage in the U.S. market.

Then, as they seemed to be on the brink of success, the company suddenly encountered a contamination problem all too reminiscent of the SV_{40} dilemma that had forced Merck out of polio vaccine production. The chick-embryo cell cultures (which had enabled researchers to stop using monkey kidney cells) were now discovered to have their own indigenous viral contaminants.[43] The appearance in the vaccine of avian leukosis (chicken leukemia) — a potentially carcinogenic virus for humans, particularly infants — threatened to derail this second major project. Hilleman immediately discussed the problem with Dr. Joseph Smadel of the Division of Biologics Standards. Smadel was not very concerned about the avian virus. As he explained, years of experience with a similarly contaminated yellow fever vaccine had produced no evidence of human carcinogenicity. Without an alternative solution, there would be no measles vaccine, with predictable results in morbidity and mortality.

But Hilleman was not convinced, and he faced the prospect of trying to convince Merck's management to take this long-term risk. Planning as they were to give shots "to many millions of healthy children," the prospect of injecting them with a leukemia virus, chicken or otherwise, made Hilleman "restive."[44] As he knew, Dr.

---

42 H. Goldner, E. B. Buynak, and M. R. Hilleman, "Infectivity Stability of Live Measles-Virus Vaccine," *American Journal of Diseases of Children* 103 (1962): 440–2. On rehydration, the dried vaccine still needed to be stored at $4°$ C. and needed to be used within one day.

43 At first this did not appear to be the case. See M. R. Hilleman and H. Goldner, "Perspectives for Testing Safety of Live Measles Vaccine," *American Journal of Diseases of Children* 103 (Mar. 1962): 489–92. As Hilleman noted, however, SV_{40} "by virtue of its failure to cause visible change in the species of monkey kidney cells in which it commonly occurs, escaped detection for many years" (p. 489).

44 M. R. Hilleman, "Past, Present, and Future of Measles, Mumps, and Rubella Virus Vaccines," *Pediatrics* 90, no. 1 (1992): 149–53.

Harry Rubin, who was then working in Nobel Laureate Wendell Stanley's laboratory at the University of California at Berkeley, had developed a test to detect avian leukosis virus.[45] Rubin had also demonstrated that hens that had leukosis virus antibodies laid eggs from which noninfected chicks were hatched. Hilleman set off in search of the fertile eggs from immune hens that would allow him to develop leukosis-free eggs. He flew to California to discuss his idea with Stanley. Stanley told him that Kimber Farms had already developed seven flocks of leukosis-free chickens. That sent Hilleman to Kimber Farms, where he found the rare experimental flocks he needed. Kimber initially had no interest in selling the chickens, but Hilleman persisted and Merck finally got the essential flocks.[46]

With the contamination problem solved, Merck Sharp & Dohme pushed ahead with the production process. The testing was more elaborate than it was for most pharmaceutical products. Because more than thirty-five separate tests had to be conducted, the company employed eight quality control scientists and technicians for every person involved in production. Under aseptic conditions, they removed the embryos from the eggs of the leukosis-free flock; they minced, washed, and trypsinized[47] the torsos to break them down into single cells. They then placed a precise number of cells in a series of carefully labeled bottles.[48] They infected about 80 percent of these cultures with measles virus that was free of all other detectable microbial contami-

---

45 This was the Resistance Inducing Factor or RIF test.

46 Convinced of the importance of the project, the research director at Kimber Farms decided to release the flocks to Merck. Hilleman's cause may have been helped by the fact that he and the research director were both from Montana, a state that apparently breeds an abiding sense of camaraderie in its citizens. M. R. Hilleman "Notes," MA. Once they obtained these flocks, the firm had a source of eggs for subsequent vaccines as well.

47 Trypsinizing involves treatment with an enzyme.

48 The labels enabled them to trace the cells back to a particular chicken if a problem should arise.

nants. The remaining cultures were left uninfected to serve as controls — a means of checking for extraneous agents. After they processed the cultures, they collected, clarified, and stored the virus-infected cell culture fluids. They later freeze-dried the pooled fluid to yield the final vaccine.

On March 22, 1963 — the day after the government announced that it had licensed the product — Merck Sharp & Dohme was ready to ship by air 100,000 doses of live-virus measles vaccine.[49] Merck's revitalized virology program had its first breakthrough product in hand and was the only firm prepared to market this vaccine.[50] Well, almost. Just as the company was gearing up for large-scale production of the vaccine — trademarked *Rubeovax* — and the standardized immune globulin — trademarked *Gammagee* — the DBS decided that there should immediately be competition in sales of the measles vaccine. Merck, which had made a large investment in building up its virology program and in developing the new product, was of course not pleased with this prospect. The DBS selected another firm's attenuated virus grown in dog kidney cell culture, but the competing product quickly proved to be so reactogenic that it had to

---

49 Hilleman, "Past, Present, and Future of Measles, Mumps, and Rubella Virus Vaccines," pp. 149–53. Press releases from MSD, West Point, Mar. 21 and 22, 1963, MA. See also the "Statement on the Status of Measles Vaccines," by the Surgeon General's Ad Hoc Advisory Committee on Measles Control, *JAMA* 183, no. 13 (1963): 120–1.

50 At this same time the government gave Chas. Pfizer & Co., of New York, a license for its inactivated vaccine, which was later removed from the market (see Note 34). *JAMA* 184, no. 2 (1963): 44. Eli Lilly & Co., was working on an inactivated vaccine and Lederle Laboratories on an attenuated live-virus vaccine. S. Karelitz, B. C. Berliner, M. Orange, S. Penbharkkul, A. Ramos, and P. Muenboon, "Inactivated Measles Virus Vaccine," *JAMA* 184, no. 9 (1963): 87–93; see pp. 135–7 in the same issue: Pitman-Moore Co., of Indianapolis, Indiana, was also working on an attenuated vaccine. On Lederle's product see also *JAMA* 177, no. 8 (1961): 67–71; and *New England Journal of Medicine* 269, no. 2 (1963): 75–7.

be removed from the market.[51] At that time Merck was thus the sole producer of the attenuated vaccine, but it had received a foretaste of some of the problems that would develop in vaccine pricing and control in future years.

Although *Rubeovax* had cleared its final hurdle, the laboratory at West Point and the clinical team from the University of Pennsylvania continued to work on improvements in the new product.[52] One that was successful was a combined measles and smallpox vaccine. Dr. Paul Grunmeier, of MSD's Biological Process Improvement Laboratories, led the effort to produce the company's first combination vaccine. His group mixed commercial batches of *Rubeovax* with sterile suspensions of calf lymph infected with vaccinia virus obtained from another firm.[53] This combination was then lyophilized and subjected to limited clinical tests (1966) that indicated it was effective in stimulating antibodies against both diseases.[54] After the DBS licensed the vaccine in 1967, Merck marketed it under the name *Dryvax*.

The following year, the government also licensed a more attenuated live measles virus vaccine that was less reactogenic. In an effort to improve *Rubeovax*, Hilleman's team had passaged the virus forty additional times in chick-embryo cell culture.[55] The work and expense involved were comparable to the effort required on *Rubeovax*.

---

51 Hilleman, "Past, Present, and Future of Measles, Mumps, and Rubella Virus Vaccines," pp. 149–53. Also, M. R. Hilleman, "Notes," MA. Chase, *Magic Shots*, pp. 312–13.

52 See also S. Krugman, S. Stone, R. Hu, and H. Friedman, "Measles Immunization Incorporated in the Routine Schedule for Infants: Efficacy of a Combined Inactivated-Live Vaccination Regime," *Pediatrics* 34, no. 6 (1964): 795–7.

53 Although Mulford and Sharp & Dohme had both produced smallpox vaccine, Merck Sharp & Dohme was not in this business.

54 R. E. Weibel, J. Stokes, Jr., E. B. Buynak, M. R. Hilleman, and P. W. Grunmeier, "Clinical-Laboratory Experiences with Combined Dried Live Measles-Smallpox Vaccine," *Pediatrics* 37, no. 6 (1966): 913–20.

55 Competitors were also working on further attenuation. *JAMA* 190, no. 8 (1964): 27–9.

Following production of the test lots, the clinical team conducted trials with about 20,000 children. Having in hand favorable results on immune response and reactogenicity, the company manufactured and clinically tested five consistency lots of the new product. The chief advantage of the resulting product – marketed as *Attenuvax* – was that it did not require immune globulin to be coadministered, greatly simplifying the task of vaccination.[56]

The measles vaccine seemed to vindicate the decision Merck management had made in 1957 to increase its investment in biologicals and to do so with new leadership in the Merck Institute. Hilleman now had in place a talented group of researchers, all of whom understood what their boss had meant when he said, "You'd better be dedicated." Working closely with the University of Pennsylvania, the Institute had developed an excellent clinical program and had established strong ties throughout the virology, pediatrics, and public health networks.[57] Determined to continue producing good science as well as innovative products, Hilleman had already launched

---

56 M. R. Hilleman, E. B. Buynak, R. E. Weibel, J. Stokes, Jr., J. E. Whitman, and M. B. Leagus, "Development and Evaluation of the Moraten Measles Virus Vaccine," *JAMA* 206, no. 3 (1968): 587-90; M. R. Hilleman, "Toward Prophylaxis of Prenatal Infection by Viruses," *Obstetrics and Gynecology* 33, no. 4 (1969): 461–9; Hilleman, "Past, Present, and Future of Measles, Mumps, and Rubella Virus Vaccines," pp. 149–53. See also R. J. Warren, P. R. Nader, and R. H. Levine, "Measles Immune Globulin," *JAMA* 203, no. 3 (1968): 120–2.

57 By 1964, pediatricians were commenting on the emerging relationships between pediatrics and virology and their respective bodies of knowledge. See H. G. Cramblett, "How Much Virology Should the Pediatrician Know?" *Pediatrics* 34, no. 6 (1964): 751–2. On public health see the *American Journal of Public Health* 52, no. 2 (1962), part 2, devoted entirely to the new measles vaccine. See also *JAMA* 188, no. 2 (1964): 150–1; and the report on the National Communicable Disease Center's Fourth Annual Immunization Conference in the *American Journal of Public Health* 57, no. 5 (1967): 921–2. For continued pediatric studies see F. A. Oski and J. L. Naiman, "Effect of Live Measles Vaccine on the Platelet Count," *New England Journal of Medicine* 275, no. 7 (1966): 352–6.

---

the Institute's program to develop a vaccine for a second major disease of childhood.

2

Mumps, known medically as *parotitis epidemica*, is an ancient endemic disease that Hippocrates described in the fifth century B.C. Like measles, it is a common childhood illness that, at its greatest severity, can cripple and kill. Ninety percent of the cases are in children under the age of fourteen, who typically display involvement of the parotid gland following fever, headaches, and malaise. The complications can include meningitis, encephalitis, impaired hearing, and at its most extreme, various neurologic syndromes. Rarely, it can even be fatal.[58]

Debate continues about other aspects of mumps. It has been associated with birth defects and juvenile diabetes. One of its most common and feared manifestations in postpubertal men is the painful epididymo-orchitis. This has prompted substantial controversy about the long-lasting effects of mumps on male fertility. In the 1960s it was thought that the disease frequently caused sterility in post-pubescent males. In the 1970s and early 1980s the medical community largely rejected this conclusion. But now again in the 1990s, the consensus has shifted: current studies indicate that approximately 13

---

58 S. G. Baum and N. Litman, "Mumps Virus," in Mandell, Douglas, and Bennett, eds., *Infectious Diseases*, pp. 1260–5. G. E. Shambaugh, E. W. Hagens, J. W. Holdrman, and R. W. Watkins, "Physical Causes of Deafness: Report of Committee, Division of Medical Sciences, National Research Council: II. Statistical Studies of the Children in the Public Schools for the Deaf," *Archives of Otolaryngology (Chicago)* 7 (1928): 424; Hilleman, "Toward Prophylaxis of Prenatal Infection by Viruses," pp. 461–9. J. P. Utz, V. N. Houk, and D. W. Alling, "Clinical and Laboratory Studies of Mumps," *New England Journal of Medicine* 270, no. 24 (1964): 1283–6; also see *New England Journal of Medicine* 271, no. 5 (1964): 251–2. C. L. Witte and B. Schanzer, "Pancreatitis Due to Mumps," *JAMA* 203, no. 12 (1968): 164–5; see also *JAMA* 209, no. 13 (1969): 2060; *Pediatrics Research* 9 (1975): 30–4; and *Pediatrics* 61, no. 1 (1978): 158.

percent of the men who have contracted the illness suffer from impaired fertility.[59]

In the 1930s, Drs. C. D. Johnson and E. W. Goodpasture had isolated the virus from the saliva of mumps patients and used it to produce the disease in monkeys. More than a decade passed, however, before researchers could grow the virus in a medium. Dr. K. Habel of the U.S. Public Health Service accomplished this in 1945, using chick-embryo cells. His work was soon picked up by Enders and his colleagues, who also cultivated the virus. In the early 1950s, there were trials with a killed-mumps-virus vaccine that could provide temporary protection.[60] But at this time, an attenuated live-virus vaccine that might give more lasting immunity still seemed out of reach.

At the Merck Institute, Hilleman and his colleagues began work on this problem in the early 1960s. As they knew, there were serious obstacles to overcome. In previous attempts, the mumps virus had lost its ability to elicit an antibody response in humans once it had been adapted to chick-embryo cultures – still the best medium to ensure sufficient attenuation. Hilleman decided to start over with a new strain of virus. He needed a wild starting virus and he found one close to home. His six-year-old daughter, Jeryl Lynn, developed clinical mumps in March 1963, and her father collected blood and saliva samples from her.[61] He and his team then isolated the *Jeryl Lynn* virus

---

59 See, for instance, R. P. Lyon and H. B. Bruyn, "Mumps Epididymo-Orchitis," *JAMA* 196, no. 8 (1966): 148–50; and Baum and Litman, "Mumps Virus," p. 1262.

60 Baum and Litman, "Mumps Virus," p. 1260; G. Henle and W. Henle, "Studies on the Prevention of Mumps," *Pediatrics* 8, no. 1 (1951): 1–4. *Merck Review* 27, no. 2 (1966). The work reported by Henle and Henle had been done by the Armed Forces Epidemiological Board and one of the collaborators was Dr. Joseph Stokes, Jr.

61 E. B. Buynak and M. R. Hilleman, "Live Attenuated Mumps Virus Vaccine: 1. Vaccine Development," *Proceedings of the Society for Experimental Biology and Medicine* 123 (1966): 768-75; Hilleman, "Past, Present, and Future of Measles,

strain by amniotic inoculation into embryonated hens' eggs collected from the leukemia-free chicken stock. Once isolated and attenuated by passage in the chick embryos, the virus was further passed in chick-embryo cell cultures.[62] After Hilleman and his coworker, Dr. Eugene Buynak, successfully attenuated this virus, they prepared several vaccines at different attenuation levels for clinical trial. Extensive laboratory testing followed, including safety and potency tests based on the standards the U.S. Public Health Service had developed for Merck's measles vaccine.[63]

The Children's Hospital/Merck clinical teams conducted the initial human trials in June 1965 on small groups of children who were injected subcutaneously with the vaccines. One of the test vaccines (using the virus after twelve passages) produced mild parotitis in a small number of the children. But another (seventeen passages) produced the desired antibody response with no parotitis or other clinical manifestations.[64]

Mumps, and Rubella Virus Vaccines," pp. 149–53; M. R. Hilleman, Interview, Nov. 13 and 21, 1991.

62 As in *Rubeovax* production, the embryos were removed from the eggs and the torsos minced, washed, and trypsinized to break the tissues into single cells. Buynak and Hilleman, "Live Attenuated Mumps Virus Vaccine: 1. Vaccine Development," pp. 768-75. *Merck Review* 27, no. 2 (1966), MA.

63 Buynak and Hilleman, "Live Attenuated Mumps Virus Vaccine: 1. Vaccine Development," pp. 768–75; J. Stokes, Jr., R. E. Weibel, E. B. Buynak, and M. R. Hilleman, "Live Attenuated Mumps Virus Vaccine: 2. Early Clinical Studies," *Pediatrics* 39, no. 3 (1967): 363–71. The dried vaccines, which were rehydrated before they were used, proved to be stable enough for clinical use.

64 As was customary at this time, the clinical team conducted the trials with institutionalized children, after the Pennsylvania Association for Retarded Children approved the tests. Stokes, Weibel, Buynak, and Hilleman, "Live Attenuated Mumps Virus Vaccine: 2. Early Clinical Studies," pp. 363–71; C. M. Martin, "Statement Before the Special Commission on Human Medical Experimentation, Commonwealth of Pennsylvania," June 1973, pp. 3–5, MA. See also *JAMA* 197, no. 2 (1966): 42.

Later, government regulations would require informed consent for clini-

Joseph Stokes and his colleague Robert E. Weibel used the latter vaccine in larger trials in 1965. The clinical and Merck teams conducted controlled field studies of 1,337 children in the Philadelphia suburbs of Havertown-Springfield.[65] The children ranged from eleven months to eleven years of age, and those with a negative history of mumps were alternately administered the vaccine or used as controls. In families with more than one child, one received the vaccine and one or more of the other children served as controls. The results of these tests and the subsequent clinical studies were favorable.[66] The vaccine was safe and effective in a single dose. It produced neither contagious infection nor significant clinical symptoms.[67] It was efficacious during a natural mumps epidemic that occurred during the Havertown-Springfield trials, and after several months had passed, the children retained their immunity.[68]

---

cal testing and eventually institutionalized persons (children or adults) would no longer be used. One of the effects of these regulations would be to send more and more clinical testing overseas.

65 All of the children had received parental consent to take part in the trials.

66 M. R. Hilleman, E. B. Buynak, R. E. Weibel, and J. Stokes, Jr., "Live Attenuated Mumps-Virus Vaccine," *New England Journal of Medicine* 278, no. 5 (1968): 227–32; see also the editorial calling for more information to justify vaccination for mumps (pp. 275–6). Twenty-five principal investigators conducted subsequent studies involving almost 6,500 seronegative children and adults.

67 Stokes, Weibel, Buynak, and Hilleman, "Live Attenuated Mumps Virus Vaccine: 2. Early Clinical Studies," pp. 363–71; R. E. Weibel, J. Stokes, Jr., E. B. Buynak, J. E. Whitman, Jr., and M. R. Hilleman, "Live Attenuated Mumps-Virus Vaccine: 3. Clinical and Serologic Aspects in Field Evaluation," *New England Journal of Medicine* 276, no. 5 (1967): 245–51; R. E. Weibel, E. B. Buynak, J. Stokes, Jr., J. E. Whitman, Jr., and M. R. Hilleman, "Evaluation of Live Attenuated Mumps Virus Vaccine, Strain Jeryl Lynn," First International Conference on Vaccines Against Viral and Rickettsial Diseases of Man, *Pan American Health Organization Scientific Publications* 147 (May 1967): 430–7. See also *JAMA* 201, no. 13 (1967): 119–22; *JAMA* 203, no. 1 (1968): 63–7 and 68–72.

68 M. R. Hilleman, R. E. Weibel, E. B. Buynak, J. Stokes, Jr., and J. E. Whitman, "Live, Attenuated Mumps-Virus Vaccine: 4. Protective Efficacy as

The government licensed Merck's product under the trade name *Mumpsvax* in 1967. Initially, the Public Health Service Advisory Committee on Immunization Practices only recommended the vaccine for use with children who were approaching puberty and older persons who had not been exposed to the disease.[69] Shortly, however, the Committee widened the guidelines to include all susceptible children over one year of age.[70] By 1969, when further clinical studies indicated that the vaccine's immunity persisted for at least three years, almost two million persons had been vaccinated with the new product.[71] After a decade of accelerated research, Merck's Virus and Cell Biology team had produced its second major innovation — and was closing in on a third.

3

Closing in, that is, amidst considerably more politicking than Merck had experienced since it left the polio vaccine business. In the 1960s, those corners of the virology network dedicated to developing a vaccine for rubella (German measles) were almost as politically charged as the polio campaign had been. In part, the politics were a product of the

Measured in a Field Evaluation," *New England Journal of Medicine* 276, no. 5 (1967): 252–8; see also the editorial on pp. 295–6.

69 *JAMA* 203, no. 4 (1968): 22. See, however, *New England Journal of Medicine* 278, no. 12 (1968): 681–2, for the more aggressive plan at the Massachusetts Department of Public Health. See also the Committee's defense of its "cautious policies" in *JAMA* 281, no. 12 (1968): 679. The debate continued in *JAMA* 281, no. 21 (1969): 1193.

70 *JAMA* 206, no. 10 (1968): 2220. The vaccine prompted the Conference of State and Territorial Epidemiologists to put mumps back on the list of notifiable diseases so that accurate data could be collected on epidemics. *JAMA* 203, no. 9 (1968): 24.

71 R. E. Weibel, E. B. Buynak, J. E. Whitman, Jr., M. B. Leagus, J. Stokes, Jr., and M. R. Hilleman, "Jeryl Lynn Strain Live Mumps Virus Vaccine," *JAMA* 207, no. 9 (1969): 1667–70. P. H. Jones, "Public Acceptance of Mumps Immunization," *JAMA* 209, no. 6 (1969): 901–5; see also *JAMA* 209, no. 13 (1969): 2042.

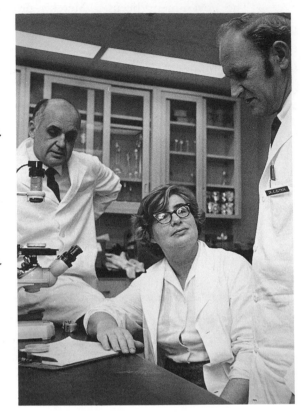

(Left to right) Dr. Maurice R. Hilleman, Executive Director of Merck's Virus and Cell Biology Research; Dr. Beverly Jean Neff, Senior Research Virologist; and Dr. Eugene B. Buynak, Director of Viral Immunology Research. 1970.

connection between this viral infection and congenital birth defects. This linkage gave unusual political salience to the efforts to control the periodic outbreaks of the disease.[72] Rubella has far more devastating congenital consequences – fetal death, heart malformation, cataracts, deafness, microcephaly, and mental retardation – than measles or mumps.[73] The relationship had been recognized at least two decades

72 Clearly, the politics of disease are not perfectly correlated with morbidity and mortality. Certain diseases elicit particularly strong public concerns, which in turn generate political support for those who are attempting to control the disease or treat afflicted persons. In the post-WWII years, public relations efforts by interested parties increasingly shaped those responses.

73 *JAMA* 175, no. 2 (1961): 158. Hilleman, "Toward Prophylaxis of Prenatal Infection by Viruses," pp. 461–9. D. I. Weiss, L. Z. Cooper, and R. H. Green,

before major efforts to prevent the disease were launched. In Australia, ophthalmologist Norman McAlister Gregg had noted the dramatic increase in the number of children born with congenital cataracts and other birth defects following the rubella epidemic of 1940–1. Gregg determined that all the affected children had been born to women who had contracted German measles during pregnancy. Although he conducted a survey and published his findings in the *Transactions of the Ophthalmological Society of Australia*, his work was largely overlooked during the all-consuming war.

During the postwar years a few scientists who had paid attention to the link between rubella and birth defects began to look for a means of immunizing pregnant women. At first they focused on conferring passive immunity by administering gamma globulin from people who had contracted the disease. In 1948, Sir Macfarlane Burnet and his coworkers successfully provided passive immunity to twenty pregnant women who had been exposed to rubella.[74] As it became clear that short-term immunity could prevent congenital birth defects, the interest in protecting women and their fetuses spread in America and abroad. Gradually, the focus shifted to an effort to develop a vaccine that would confer lasting immunity.[75]

Isolation of the virus – the necessary first step – proved to be an extremely difficult task that confounded even John Enders. But in this case one of Enders's students, Thomas Weller, was able to surpass his mentor. In 1952 Weller had become professor of tropical medicine

"Infantile Glaucoma," *JAMA* 195, no. 9 (1966): 105–7. See also C. S. Karmody, "Subclinical Maternal Rubella and Congenital Deafness," *New England Journal of Medicine* 278, no. 15 (1968): 809–14; also see *New England Journal of Medicine* 292, no. 19 (1975): 1023–4. H. Stern, S. D. Elek, J. C. Booth, D. G. Fleck, "Microbial Causes of Mental Retardation," *Lancet* (Aug. 30, 1969): 443–8.

74 T. C. Doege and K. S. W. Kim, "Studies of Rubella and Its Prevention with Immune Globulin," *JAMA* 200, no. 7 (1967): 104–10. *Lancet* (Sept. 6, 1969): 546.

75 F. L. Babbott, Jr., B. M. Rodenberger, and T. H. Ingalls, "Rubella," *JAMA* 178, no. 6 (1961): 128–32. Chase, *Magic Shots*, p. 315.

at the Harvard School of Public Health. He concentrated his research on the main endemic, infectious disease killers of the tropics: measles, mumps, and rubella. He became especially concerned with rubella in 1960, when his ten-year-old son contracted an unusually severe case of the disease. That same year the U.S. Army also became worried when a rubella epidemic broke out among the new recruits at Fort Dix, New Jersey. At that time, both Weller and an Army research group (led by Paul Parkman, E. L. Buescher, and Malcolm S. Artenstein, of the Walter Reed Army Institute of Research) were able to isolate the virus.[76]

This left a vaccine in reach, but tragically the next epidemic came before one could be developed. In 1963–5, the United States suffered one of its worst outbreaks of rubella.[77] Although the disease was poorly tracked and underreported, it was estimated to have caused at least 20,000 fetal deaths. This epidemic alone afflicted another 20,000 children with prenatal brain damage.[78] The resulting public anguish

---

76 T. H. Weller and F. A. Neva, "Propagation in Tissue Culture of Cytopathic Agents from Patients with Rubella-like Illness," *Proceedings of the Society for Experimental Biology and Medicine* 8 (1962): 215–25; in the same volume see P. D. Parkman, E. L. Bueschner, and M. S. Artenstein, "Recovery of Rubella Virus from Army Recruits," pp. 225–30. *New England Journal of Medicine* 267, no. 22 (1962): 1153. In 1960 Hilleman introduced at Merck the subject of a rubella vaccine, even though the disease still had an "unknown etiology." M. R. Hilleman to M. Tishler, July 5, 1960, MA. Hilleman regarded Artenstein's isolation of the virus as the most practical one. M. R. Hilleman, "Notes," MA.

77 C. A. Phillips, A. M. Behbehani, L. W. Johnson, and J. L. Melnick, "Isolation of Rubella Virus," *JAMA* 191, no. 8 (1965): 79–82; see also pp. 83–90. Chase, *Magic Shots*, p. 316; and *JAMA* 191, no. 10 (1965): 139–41, 148–9.

78 J. E. Banatvala, D. M. Horstmann, M. C. Payne, and L. Gluck, "Rubella Syndrome and Thrombocytopenic Purpura in Newborn Infants," *New England Journal of Medicine* 273, no. 9 (1965): 474–8. R. Achs, R. G. Harper, and M. Siegel, "Unusual Dermatoglyphic Findings Associated with Rubella Embryopathy," *New England Journal of Medicine* 274, no. 3 (1966): 148–50. J. Stokes,

---

prompted a public effort to prevent the disease. The widespread concern lent further support to those who were urging Congress to approve Title XIX (the Medicaid provisions) of the Social Security Act of 1965. Congress responded with the Early and Periodic Screening, Diagnosis, and Treatment amendments to Title XIX, mandating the right of every American child to receive comprehensive pediatric care, including vaccinations.

When Congress passed and President Johnson signed the new law, it was in part a consequence of the mounting public anxiety about the degree of vaccination in general and the protection from rubella in particular. The new policy was poorly administered and even ignored by many states, but it laid a foundation for the mass immunization programs that were to follow in the United States.[79] There was strong interest in having a program for German measles, and since rubella usually built up to epidemic levels every six to nine years, the research and development programs then underway at Merck and at the DBS were under substantial pressure to produce results quickly. It was fairly certain there would be another epidemic in the 1970s, probably early in the decade.[80]

Hilleman's team of scientists and their clinical collaborators in Philadelphia had been working on rubella for two years. In 1962, Buynak and Hilleman had isolated the Benoit strain of the virus.[81] Given the menacing shadow of the next epidemic, they decided first to develop a killed-virus vaccine. While it would only confer temporary immunity, it could, they thought, be produced and tested quickly. By

---

Jr., R. E. Weibel, E. B. Buynak, and M. R. Hilleman, "Protective Efficacy of Duck Embryo Rubella Vaccines," *Pediatrics* 44, no. 2 (1969): 217–24.

79 Chase, *Magic Shots*, pp. 316–17.

80 M. R. Hilleman, E. B. Buynak, R. E. Weibel, and J. Stokes, Jr., "Live Attenuated Rubella-Virus Vaccine," *New England Journal of Medicine* 279, no. 6 (1968): 300–3.

81 The name, as usual, was provided by the person whose sample provided the virus, in this case a Philadelphia schoolboy named Benoit.

1965, however, they had decided to abandon that route – as had the DBS – and focus only on a live-virus vaccine.[82]

Their first major problem was to find an appropriate growth medium for propagating and attenuating the virus. Chick-embryo cells were not susceptible to the virus.[83] Realizing that rubella virus did the most damage in the first trimester of pregnancy, Hilleman decided that it might prefer less differentiated cells for propagation. Knowing that duck embryos are less differentiated than those of chicks at the same age, he tried this approach. Whether the reasoning was right or not, the experiment worked, providing an effective medium. Virus and Cell Biology prepared for testing a number of vaccines that had gone through different numbers of passages.[84] By January 1965, they were able to attenuate the Benoit strain of the virus rapidly and dependably for use in humans.[85] Meanwhile, the team at DBS had been working with bovine kidney cells and had passaged a different strain of the virus

82 J. Stokes, Jr., R. E. Weibel, E. B. Buynak, and M. R. Hilleman, "Clinical and Laboratory Tests of Merck Strain Live Attenuated Rubella Virus Vaccine," First International Conference on Vaccines Against Viral and Rickettsial Diseases of Man, *Pan American Health Organization Scientific Publications* 147 (May 1967): 402–5. See also A. D. Heggie, "Rubella: Current Concepts in Epidemiology and Teratology," *Pediatric Clinics of North America* 13, no. 2 (1966): 251–66.

83 A. Reddick and C. E. Roesel, "Rubella Virus: Growth and Cytopathic Effect in Primary Cultures of Cells of Rabbit Embryos," *Science* 151 (Mar. 18, 1966): 1405–6, reports on the various efforts to solve this problem.

84 E. B. Buynak, M. R. Hilleman, R. E. Weibel, and J. Stokes, Jr., "Live Attenuated Rubella Virus Vaccines Prepared in Duck Embryo Cell Culture: I. Development and Clinical Testing," *JAMA* 204, no. 3 (1968): 103–8. Ducks are relatively disease-free and were found to contain no extraneous viruses. M. R. Hilleman, E. B. Buynak, J. E. Whitman, Jr., R. E. Weibel, and J. Stokes, Jr., "Live Attenuated Rubella Virus Vaccines: Experience with Duck Embryo Cell Preparations," *American Journal of the Diseases of Children* 118 (Aug. 1969): 166–71.

85 *JAMA* 196, no. 6 (1966): 25–6, reported on the progress being made by the NIH and the Merck/Penn teams. Hilleman, "Past, Present, and Future of Measles, Mumps, and Rubella Virus Vaccines," pp. 149–53; M. R. Hilleman, Interview, Nov. 13 and 21, 1991.

seventy-seven times (HPV-77). By 1966, Paul Parkman had collaborated with Dr. Harry Meyer, Jr., and Theodore C. Panos to produce an attenuated live-rubella-virus vaccine that they had tested on animals and small groups of children. Merck was also pushing ahead with clinical research on its vaccine.[86]

Both Merck and the DBS were thus making significant progress when Mary Lasker intervened and transformed a scientific horserace into a complex, multisided political struggle. Lasker was, by dint of the Albert and Mary Lasker Foundation, a prominent promoter of medical science and an influential health lobbyist.[87] She expressed to Hilleman and his Merck colleagues her fear that competition between the two laboratories might impede the pace of vaccine development and introduction. The two groups, she said, should concentrate on a single virus. She explained that she favored the DBS (HPV-77) virus for what were essentially political reasons: she thought that the biologics division might act more expeditiously if its own virus were chosen. Others were concerned as well, including the Vaccine Development Board of the National Institute of Allergy and Infectious Diseases (NIAID), which had promised the nation an effective vaccine by 1970. NIAID's reputation was on the line.[88]

---

86 P. D. Parkman, H. M. Meyer, Jr., R. L. Kirschstein, and H. E. Hopps, "Attenuated Rubella Virus: I. Development and Laboratory Characterization," and H. M. Meyer, Jr., P. D. Parkman, and T. C. Panos, "Attenuated Rubella Virus: II. Production of an Experimental Live-Virus Vaccine and Clinical Trial," both in *New England Journal of Medicine* 275, no. 11 (1966): 569–74 and 575–80, respectively; see also the editorial (pp. 615–16), which comments on the progress of the Penn/Merck team. Stokes, Weibel, Buynak, and Hilleman, "Clinical and Laboratory Tests of Merck Strain Live Attenuated Rubella Virus Vaccine," pp. 402–5. M. R. Hilleman, "Notes," MA. See also *Lancet* (Feb. 4, 1967): 261–2.

87 Shorter, *The Health Century*, pp. 56–7, 204–5, 241.

88 M. R. Hilleman, "Summary of Clinical and Laboratory Tests of Merck Strain and of Meyer-Parkman HPV-77 Live Attenuated Rubella Virus Vaccines Grown in Cell Cultures of Duck Embryo," Sept. 29, 1967; M. R. Hilleman to Daniel Mullally, Oct. 3, 1967; M. R. Hilleman to Max Tishler, Sept. 29, 1967; M. R.

But as the Merck scientists fully understood, status in the virology and pediatrics networks and in the larger society would flow to the party whose virus was employed in the final product. Commercially, it was a toss-up. Here, then, was the sort of struggle that would become common in these networks during the next few decades: in this case and others, science yielded to politics and commerce. Displaying "ethical constraint," Hilleman and his colleagues decided to work with both of the viruses.[89] When their clinical tests demonstrated that the HPV-77 virus was too toxic for routine use, they further attenuated it in duck-embryo cell culture. Their studies now indicated that the Benoit and "HPV-77 duck" viruses were equally effective and acceptably reactogenic, so they moved ahead with the latter virus.[90]

The Penn/Merck teams quickly expanded the clinical trials, even though these tests for safety and efficacy created complex liability problems for the company. The vaccination of children might constitute a hazard (teratogenicity) to pregnant women to whom the virus could be transmitted. Even if this did not happen, the firm could be blamed for congenital defects of the sort that occur in 3 percent of births. Apprehensive but determined to continue developing its new product and its capability in biologicals, Merck bit the bullet and went to the next stage of testing. By this time, there was pressure from a medical community fearful that the vaccine still might not be ready before the next epidemic.[91]

The clinical teams conducted large-scale tests in various insti-

---

Hilleman to Those Concerned, Oct. 3, 1967; M. R. Hilleman to J. Fletcher, Apr. 21, 1972; all in MA.

89 M. R. Hilleman, Interview, Nov. 13 and 21, 1991.

90 M. R. Hilleman to Leonard Hayflick, Apr. 21, 1972, with enclosures, MA. Hilleman recalls that he talked to Dr. Meyer of the DBS about the element of scientific sacrifice involved in this decision. Meyer, he said, agreed. M. R. Hilleman, "Notes," MA. The Merck group salvaged some status by adding "duck" to "HPV-77."

91 JAMA 200, no. 9 (1967): 37; 202, no. 7 (1967): 42; 203, no. 5 (1968): 22.

tutions and among families in the same Philadelphia area that had participated in the measles and mumps studies. They administered the vaccine subcutaneously, with promising results.[92] At least 97 percent of the 265 susceptible children in the community who received the vaccine developed rubella antibodies without causing their contact siblings or susceptible mothers to produce antibodies. There were no clinical symptoms. Merck now concluded that it had another safe, effective vaccine, and Meyer and Parkman later confirmed these findings.[93]

Given these results, the company pushed ahead with more extensive clinical tests.[94] In the spring of 1968, Dr. R. W. McCollum of Yale administered the vaccine to 2,600 children in Danbury, Connecticut, during the peak of a German-measles outbreak in that area. No new cases of the disease developed among those who received the vaccine, while unvaccinated children continued to succumb. Dr.

92 Hilleman, "Toward Prophylaxis of Prenatal Infection by Viruses," pp. 465–6. The Merck team determined from the data that the virus actually had to be excreted by the vaccine recipient in order to have achieved adequate immunity. It was imperative, however, that excreted virus not be contagious, and they achieved that goal in the clinical tests.

93 Buynak, Hilleman, Weibel, and Stokes, "Live Attenuated Rubella Virus Vaccines Prepared in Duck Embryo Cell Culture: I. Development and Clinical Testing," pp. 103–8; and R. E. Weibel, J. Stokes, Jr., E. B. Buynak, J. E. Whitman, Jr., M. B. Leagus, and M. R. Hilleman, "Live Attenuated Rubella Virus Vaccines Prepared in Duck Embryo Cell Culture: II. Clinical Tests in Families and in an Institution," *JAMA* 205, no. 8 (1968): 82–6. Hilleman, Buynak, Weibel, and Stokes, "Live, Attenuated Rubella-Virus Vaccine," pp. 300–3. M. R. Hilleman, E. B. Buynak, J. E. Whitman, Jr., R. E. Weibel, and J. Stokes, Jr., "Summary Report on Rubella Virus Vaccines Prepared in Duck Embryo Cell Culture," and J. Stokes, Jr., R. E. Weibel, E. B. Buynak, and M. R. Hilleman, "Clinical-Laboratory Findings in Adult Women Given HPV-77 Rubella Vaccine," both in *International Symposium on Rubella Vaccines* (Basel, 1969), pp. 349–56 and 415–22, respectively.

94 See the review in H. M. Meyer, Jr., P. D. Parkman, and H. E. Hopps, "The Control of Rubella," *Pediatrics* 44, no. 1 (1969): 5–23.

Joseph Pagono also conducted extensive trials in North Carolina, as did Dr. Victor Villarejos in Costa Rica, and the National Institute of Allergy and Infectious Diseases (NIAID) in Taiwan.[95] An international conference on rubella immunization (1968 in London) prepared the ground for DBS licensing of the Merck vaccine the following year.[96] Meanwhile, the company had waiting in the wings a flock of Pekin ducks to produce fertile eggs for propagating the virus for the new vaccine. Anticipating a large and immediate demand, Merck had 600,000 doses ready for release when the DBS announced its favorable decision.[97]

Even though *Meruvax* was now licensed, Merck conducted additional clinical studies. It was crucial in this case that reactogenicity be acceptable and that attenuation be optimal to ensure that durable

---

95 See *JAMA* 206, no. 6 (1968): 1195; and 207, no. 6 (1969): 1107–10. Also G. L. Gitnick, D. A. Fuccillo, J. L. Sever, and R. J. Huebner, "Progress in Rubella Vaccine Development," *American Journal of Public Health* 58, no. 7 (1968): 1237–47. Hilleman, Buynak, Whitman, Weibel, and Stokes, "Live Attenuated Rubella Virus Vaccines," pp. 166–71; see also *American Journal of Diseases of Children* 118 (1969): 347–54. Stokes, Weibel, Buynak, and Hilleman, "Protective Efficacy of Duck Embryo Rubella Vaccines," pp. 217–24.

Merck had for some time been extending its clinical testing network, and Hilleman was personally responsible for recruiting the new scientists. Clinical research was greatly facilitated by affiliating with the International Center for Medical Research and Training, Louisiana State University School of Medicine in San Jose, Costa Rica (under the direction of Dr. Villarejos). Merck supported this liaison with personnel and equipment, and it became the means of rapidly conducting massive clinical tests in Costa Rica, Honduras, and Guatemala.

96 *JAMA* 208, no. 11 (1969): 2004. Merck planned to have two million doses ready by Aug. 1.

97 Ibid. The second company to receive a license was Philips Roxane Laboratories, Inc., Columbus, Ohio. For six months, however, Merck was the only company with a licensed product. Smith, Kline and French Laboratories, Philadelphia (SKF) had a vaccine licensed in Switzerland, Belgium, West Germany, Australia, South Africa, and Mexico in 1969. *JAMA* 207, no. 4 (1969): 709–12; 207, no. 5 (1969): 848; 210, no. 2 (1969): 342; and 210, no. 12 (1969): 2169-70. *Merck Review* 30, no. 2 (1969). The ducks were kept under a special quarantine.

immunity would be maintained through childbearing age. Judging from the previous clinical trials, the initial level of vaccine attenuation was excessively reactogenic in adult women. In a high proportion, it produced fevers, rashes (which were absent in children), arthritis, and arthralgia. It was not only the strains of HPV-77 grown in duck-embryo cultures that produced arthritis. Other researchers discovered similar symptoms with HPV-77 grown in dog-kidney and rabbit-kidney cultures.[98]

Additional investigations with HPV-77 explored the relationship between the patient's age and the occurrence of arthritis.[99] These studies indicated that children under the age of twelve did not develop joint reactions, that about 7.5 percent of the twelve to twenty-five year olds developed some joint problems, and that almost 60 percent of women between ages twenty-six and forty-one experienced arthritis or arthralgia. While these reactions were of limited duration without sequelae, they suggested that vaccination should take place at an early age, and certainly before the age of twenty-six.[100] The federal government adopted a successful vaccination policy consistent with these

---

98 R. E. Weibel, J. Stokes, Jr., E. B. Buynak, and M. R. Hilleman, "Rubella Vaccination in Adult Females," *New England Journal of Medicine* 280, no. 13 (1969): 682–5. *JAMA* 210, no. 12 (1969): 2169–70. See also V. M. Villarejos, J. A. Arguedas, G. C. Hernandez, E. B. Buynak, and M. R. Hilleman, "Clinical Laboratory Evaluation of Rubella Virus Vaccine Given to Postpartum Women Without Pregnancy Preventive," *Obstetrics and Gynecology* 42, no. 5 (1973): 689–95.

99 Stokes, Weibel, Buynak, and Hilleman, "Clinical-Laboratory Findings in Adult Women Given HPV-77 Rubella Vaccine," pp. 415–22; Stokes, Weibel, Buynak, and Hilleman, "Protective Efficacy of Duck Embryo Rubella Vaccines," pp. 217–24.

100 R. E. Weibel, J. Stokes, Jr., E. B. Buynak, and M. R. Hilleman, "Influence of Age on Clinical Response to HPV-77 Duck Rubella Vaccine," *JAMA* 222, no. 7 (1972): 805–7. See also *JAMA* 213, no. 6 (1970): 1040. Later, Dr. Stanley Plotkin would introduce the RA 27/3 strain, which produced fewer cases of arthropathy in adult women. Hilleman, "Past, Present, and Future of Measles, Mumps, and Rubella Virus Vaccines," pp. 149–53.

findings. Federal policy focused on achieving vaccination of most infants and young children in an effort to reduce the reservoir of rubella virus in the population. If successful, pregnant women in this country would seldom be exposed to the virus.[101]

In 1969, immunization teams in Laconia, New Hampshire, launched the first community-wide application of Merck's *Meruvax*. Armed with the vaccine and jet guns, they spent five days covering the town's sixteen schools. Those involved with the program had a powerful sense of urgency because of the threat of a rubella epidemic in the next few years. Other public health education campaigns followed, and by the early 1970s the results of these efforts were apparent.[102]

The long-feared epidemic never took place. By 1972 the number of reported cases of rubella had dropped from 57,686 (1969) to 25,501.[103] Thirteen million Americans had been vaccinated, two million of them by private physicians and the rest by public health workers. As a result, reported cases of German measles in the United States fell to 11,795 by 1979.[104]

---

101 S. A. Plotkin, "Rubella Vaccine," in Stanley A. Plotkin and Edward A. Mortimer, Jr., eds., *Vaccines*, 2nd edition (Philadelphia, 1994), pp. 319–23. As the author notes (p. 321), "since the licensing of the vaccine in 1969, no major epidemic of rubella has occurred, despite the previously observed six- to nine-year cycle."

102 J. A. Veronelli, "An Open Community Trial of Live Rubella Vaccines," *JAMA* 213, no. 11 (1970): 1829–36. R. P. Lipman, M. B. Bethel, J. H. Wooten, R. H. Levine, and J. S. Pagano, "Attenuated Rubella Vaccine (HPV-77): Evaluation in a Large Controlled Trial," *American Journal of Public Health* 61, no. 7 (1971): 1392–1402. Also see *JAMA* 211, no. 5 (1970): 758; 212, no. 12 (1970): 2043; 213, no. 1 (1970): 23–4; 213, no. 11 (1970): 1904–5.

103 By Oct. 1969, Merck had already shipped 2.2 million doses of the new vaccine. *JAMA* 210, no. 2 (1969): 233. In 1970 the company sold almost 13.6 million doses of *Meruvax*. J. F. Modlin, A. D. Brandling-Bennett, J. J. Witte, C. C. Campbell, and J. D. Meyers, "A Review of Five Years' Experience with Rubella Vaccine in the United States," *Pediatrics* 55, no. 1 (1975): 20–9.

104 *JAMA* 213, no. 1 (1970): 24. *Merck Review* (1970); Chase, *Magic Shots*, p. 317.

4

Despite the success with *Meruvax*, neither Merck nor the government could afford to neglect the central problem in this area of public health: persuading large numbers of parents to have their children properly vaccinated. Merck had begun to deal with this problem shortly after the government approved *Rubeovax*, its measles vaccine. In 1964 the company launched a large-scale marketing campaign for this new product. "Measles Only Gave Her Spots — Will Your Child Be As Lucky?" was MSD's message to the American public that year.[105] The company ran full-page advertisements in such popular magazines as *McCall's, Parents, Today's Health, Good Housekeeping, Redbook,* and *Family Circle.*[106] Within a few years, this campaign, the public health and practitioner support for vaccination, and the state requirements for immunization before children could be admitted to school had made deep inroads into the resistance to immunization.[107] By 1969, Hilleman was able to report in *Science* magazine that in this country measles had been "reduced . . . to trivial importance."[108]

Similar results were achieved with *Mumpsvax*. Within one year of its introduction in 1967, Merck sold 1,961,811 doses of the new vaccine. The company sold more than eleven million doses in the first five years, and the effects were quickly apparent.[109] This was true even though there were no mass immunization campaigns and mumps vaccination did

105 Press release, West Point, Nov. 5, 1964, MA.

106 Ibid.

107 See, for instance, H. D. Riley, Jr., "Current Concepts in Immunization," *Pediatric Clinics of North America* 13, no. 1 (1966): 75–104. *JAMA* 197, no. 6 (1966): 41. *New England Journal of Medicine* 289, no. 15 (1973): 811; 294, no. 26 (1976): 1459–61. *American Journal of Public Health* 67, no. 8 (1977): 763–4.

108 M. R. Hilleman, "Toward Control of Viral Infections in Man," *Science* 164 (May 2, 1969): 509. Much later, the immunization problem would reemerge in this country.

109 Attachment to memo from J. D. Phillips, "Live Virus Vaccine Usage Since Introduction," Jan. 16, 1973, MA.

not take priority over other "more essential" public health efforts.[110] As a result of vaccination, the number of reported cases of mumps in the United States declined from 185,691 to 59,647 by 1975.[111]

Favorable as these statistics were, the company and public health officials knew that without continued efforts to encourage vaccination, backsliding was likely to occur. Once a disease seemed to be "conquered" − military language has always been popular where efforts to cope with disease are involved − parents were likely to become lax about getting their children's shots.[112] One of the ways to improve

---

110 *Pediatrics* 43 (1969): 907−9. *New England Journal of Medicine* 289, no. 23 (1973): 1255. G. F. Hayden, S. R. Preblud, W. A. Orenstein, and J. L. Conrad, "Current Status of Mumps and Mumps Vaccine in the United States," *Pediatrics* 62, no. 6 (1978): 965−9.

111 Baum and Litman, "Mumps Virus," p. 1260. D. R. Arday, D. D. Kanjarpane, and P. W. Kelley, "Mumps in the U.S. Army 1980−86: Should Recruits Be Immunized?" *American Journal of Public Health* 79, no. 4 (1989): 471−4. In 1976, it was estimated that slightly less than half of the nation's one- to nine-year-old population had been vaccinated. In this case, too, there would later be immunization problems.

112 In 1966 and 1967, a combination of federal, state, and local public health authorities and professional organizations launched a large-scale campaign to eradicate measles in the United States. *JAMA* 198, no. 7 (1966): 47; 198, no. 8 (1966): 35. *Journal of Public Health* 57, no. 5 (1967): 729−30. In a two-year period, about 14 million doses of vaccine were administered. *JAMA* 203, no. 5 (1968): 21−2. *New England Journal of Medicine* 279, no. 15 (1968): 783−9. But the campaign encountered problems in ghetto areas in American cities. *JAMA* 209, no. 2 (1969): 191−2. And by the 1970s, vaccination rates had stabilized and the number of reported cases of measles had increased. *American Journal of Public Health* 64, no. 10 (1974): 939−44. In the mid-1970s, the CDC designated immunization action months in an effort to cope with the problem. *Pediatrics* 52, no. 4 (1973): 483−4; 56, no. 4 (1975): 493−4. *American Journal of Public Health* 64, no. 10 (1974): 1008, 1111−12.

A similar situation would develop with mumps in the 1980s. There would be a resurgence of the disease in 1986 and 1987, and the AAP would recommend a second dose of the vaccine. The problem would apparently stem from the failure of parents to have their children vaccinated. Baum and Litman, "Mumps Virus," p. 1260.

vaccination rates and prevent backsliding was to simplify the immunization procedures.

Merck tried to do that by developing combined vaccines, so that there would be fewer visits to the doctor and fewer shots.[113] The company had already accomplished this goal with the measles and smallpox vaccines, and now it sought to combine *Meruvax* and *Mumpsvax* with the measles vaccine.[114] There were several major hurdles to clear. Hilleman and his teams had to ensure that the different vaccines did not interfere with each other in competition for host immune responses. They also had to be concerned that the combination did not collectively increase reactogenicity beyond the level encountered when the vaccines were given individually. A combination vaccine also posed problems for quality control, because the potency of each component had to be certified for each combined lot.[115]

The result of this effort was a trivalent combination of the

---

113 Hilleman, "Past, Present, and Future of Measles, Mumps, and Rubella Virus Vaccines," pp. 149–53. It was also possible that a Merck product would be squeezed out of the market by the widespread use of another firm's combination vaccine. Merck did not have a DPT combination, and there were efforts in the 1960s to combine DPT and measles vaccinations. *American Journal of Public Health* 50, no. 10 (1960): 1529–38; 55, no. 11 (1965): 1813–19. *Pediatrics* 30 (1962): 720–36. *JAMA* 186, no. 6 (1963): 533–6; 191, no. 13 (1965): 89–92. On some of the problems that developed see *Pediatrics* 32 (1963): 446. *JAMA* 186, no. 6 (1963): 144–5. *Lancet* (Aug. 20, 1966): 424–5.

114 E. B. Buynak, R. E. Weibel, J. E. Whitman, Jr., J. Stokes, Jr., and M. R. Hilleman, "Combined Live Measles, Mumps, and Rubella Virus Vaccines," *JAMA* 207, no. 12 (1969): 2259–62. After the development of *Attenuvax*, they used this vaccine for the measles component. Later, they used Dr. Stanley Plotkin's RA 27/3 rubella in the combination. See also M. A. Budd, R. G. Scholtens, R. F. McGehee, Jr., and P. Gardner, "An Evaluation of Measles and Smallpox Vaccines Simultaneously Administered," *American Journal of Public Health* 57, no. 1 (1967): 80–6.

115 The Hilleman team solved this latter problem by selective neutralization of two of the components, allowing growth only of the third. By conducting three tests, they were able to assay each of the components specifically.

---

measles, *Jeryl Lynn* mumps, and modified HPV-77 duck-embryo rubella vaccines. Faculty members and researchers at the University of Pennsylvania Medical School's Department of Pediatrics conducted extensive clinical tests on the new vaccine, which was used only among children who had neither contracted nor been vaccinated for any of the three diseases. These trials involved elaborate studies of compatibility and different dosage adjustments, as well as efforts to establish consistent standards of clinical performance. As the Philadelphia area tests indicated, the immune reactions and reactogenicity were not significantly different than to any of the three vaccines separately. When these tests were completed, the government licensed *M-M-R* in 1971.[116]

While working on *M-M-R*, Merck's vaccine team also came up with a variety of other combinations for use in specific target groups: these included measles-mumps (*M-M-Vax*), measles-rubella (*M-R-Vax*), and mumps-rubella (*Biavax*). In each of these combinations, they used the most up-to-date virus vaccines the firm had developed.[117] Hilleman, Merck's management, and public health officials in the United States and overseas had ample reason to be pleased with the combination vaccines.[118]

---

116 Buynak, Weibel, Whitman, Stokes, and Hilleman, "Combined Live Measles, Mumps, and Rubella Virus Vaccines," pp. 2259–62; see also *JAMA* 206, no. 3 (1968): 498. Hilleman, "Toward Prophylaxis of Prenatal Infection by Viruses," pp. 461–9. M. R. Hilleman, R. E. Weibel, V. M. Villarejos, E. B. Buynak, J. Stokes, Jr., J. A. Arguedas G., and G. Vargas, "Combined Live Virus Vaccines," *Pan American Health Organization Scientific Publications* 226 (1971): 397–400. See also J. M. Borgono, R. Greiber, G. Solari, F. Concha, B. Carrillo, and M. R. Hilleman, "A Field Trial of Combined Measles-Mumps-Rubella Vaccine," *Clinical Pediatrics* 12, no. 3 (1973): 170–2; and C. F. Phillips, "Children Out of Step with Immunization," *Pediatrics* 55, no. 6 (1975): 877–81.

117 Hilleman, "Past, Present, and Future of Measles, Mumps, and Rubella Virus Vaccines," pp. 149–53. See also Note 13 in this chapter, and *JAMA* 213, no. 11 (1970): 1774.

118 The company awarded Hilleman his first Merck Directors' Scientific Award in 1969. For Merck, *M-M-R* became the "work horse" vaccine (Hilleman's words).

During these years, Merck became involved for the first time with international public health programs.[119] International organizations were just beginning to extend immunization into parts of the Third World that had rudimentary health systems and very little income to support preventive medicine.[120] Prior to licensure (1963) of *Rubeovax*, Dr. Harry Meyer of DBS used this vaccine for large-scale measles immunizations in Upper Volta (now Burkina Faso) in old French West Africa. After the DBS licensed the vaccine, the U.S. Agency for International Development (AID) supported Merck's measles immunization plan in West Africa. Merck furnished the vaccines, trucks, equipment, and personnel, while AID compensated the firm for the field operation. Working with a French West African health federation, the project (directed by Dr. F. Kalabus of the Canadian Public Health Service) conducted large-scale immunization programs throughout the region.[121]

Later, the company tested its new measles-smallpox combination vaccine in Upper Volta, under the sponsorship of the country's Ministry of Health. Dr. Kalabus again directed the successful field study, which involved 18,000 children. From a public health perspective, the combination vaccine had important logistical and economic

---

119 The bulk of the company's sales of vaccines were in the U.S. market. There were significant public policy barriers and stiff competition from national firms blocking entry into European markets. H. Lipmanowicz, *Vaccine Study – 1979*, MA. In the United Kingdom, authorities were slow to adopt mass vaccination, and Merck products faced competition from Glaxo and Wellcome. *Lancet* (June 1, 1963): 1208; *Lancet* (Aug. 14, 1965): 317–18; *Lancet* (Feb. 24, 1968): 410–12; *Lancet* (July 5, 1969): 55–6. But also see *Lancet* (Aug. 10, 1974): 326–7.

120 W. C. Cockburn, "The Programme of the World Health Organization in Medical Virology," *Progress in Medical Virology* 6 (1964): 175–92; and 15 (1973): 159–204.

121 *JAMA* 184, no. 2 (1963): 44; and 189, no. 12 (1964): 978. See also Budd, Scholtens, McGehee, and Gardner, "An Evaluation of Measles and Smallpox Vaccines Simultaneously Administered," pp. 80–6.

advantages in a setting where it was difficult to administer any large-scale health plan.[122]

From the vantage point of the early 1970s, the performance of Merck's vaccine operations was excellent and the outlook promising. There was mounting competition among the small number of successful vaccine producers in the United States.[123] But by this time, Hilleman's Virus and Cell Biology operation had become the leading innovator in the industry. Indeed, the pace of innovation in the firm was quickening near the end of the 1960s, and between 1968 and 1972, the firm sold almost sixty-one million doses of the new vaccines for measles, mumps, and rubella.[124]

This new capability was all the more important because the firm was nearing the end of a long cycle of successful innovation in medicinal chemistry. From the late 1930s through the 1960s, Merck's growth had been sustained by a series of new products discovered through screening, assays, chemical isolation, and chemical synthesis. The company's major new products had included important vitamins, antibiotics, anti-inflammatories, and antihypertensive medicines. But

---

122 F. Kalabus, H. Sansarricq, P. Lambin, J. Proulx, and M. R. Hilleman, "Standardization and Mass Application of Combined Live Measles-Smallpox Vaccine in Upper Volta," *American Journal of Epidemiology* 86, no. 1 (1967): 93–111.

123 Part of this competition took place by way of clinical trials. Talented clinical teams combined with astute management of the vaccine enterprise thus became a competitive weapon in the struggle for market share in biologicals. For examples of how this worked, compare the following studies: Measles: *Pediatrics* 36, no. 1 (1965): 40–50; 37, no. 4 (1966): 649–65. *JAMA* 189, no. 10 (1964): 723–8; 190, no. 11 (1964): 91–4; 199, no. 9 (1967): 619–23. *American Journal of Public Health* 56, no. 11 (1966): 1891–7; 57, no. 8 (1967): 1333–40. *Lancet* (Aug. 6, 1966): 345–6. *New England Journal of Medicine* 280, no. 12 (1969): 628–33. In rubella, the contests were even more spirited: *American Journal of Public Health* 61, no. 1 (1971): 152–6. *Pediatrics* 47, no. 1 (1971): 7–15. *JAMA* 211, no. 6 (1970): 991–5. *New England Journal of Medicine* 285, no. 24 (1971): 1333–9.

124 "Live Virus Vaccines: Net Doses Sold Since Introduction," enclosed with J. D. Phillips to Mr. Beck, et al., Jan. 16, 1973, MA. H. Lipmanowicz, *Vaccine Study – 1979*, MA.

in the early 1970s the pace of innovation was slowing at the Merck Sharp & Dohme Research Laboratories.

This sea change in research made the innovations in vaccines all the more important. Before 1953, Merck had not been involved with biologicals, and after the merger with Sharp & Dohme, vaccines had continued to be a negligible factor in the firm's expansion for almost fifteen years. But by the end of the 1960s, the vaccine business began to make an important contribution to the income sheet at Merck Sharp & Dohme. In 1969, vaccine products accounted for three-fifths of MSD's growth in sales. They contributed four-ninths in the following year.[125] These were the kind of figures that caught the eye of top management. In slightly more than a decade, Hilleman and his teams had logged significant advances in the control of three major diseases of children and had transformed Merck into one of the leading players in the domestic market for vaccines.

The Merck Sharp & Dohme Research Laboratories had given Hilleman and the Virus and Cell Biology research teams an unusual degree of autonomy, and after some initial disappointments, the vaccine operations had justified Merck's investment and support. Taking a long-term view, Merck had in effect prepared itself for a downturn in medicinal chemistry's long cycle of innovation. The research administrators who supported Virus and Cell Biology through this transition were organic chemists and their positions of authority had been achieved during medicinal chemistry's heyday. So too with the corporate executives, especially CEOs John Connor, Henry Gadsden, and John Horan. All had been able to see beyond their own careers and ensure that the corporation would have the new capabilities needed to carry it through this transformation. For executives and science administrators in a modern corporation, there is no more important responsibility.

125 H. Lipmanowicz, *Vaccine Study – 1979*, MA.

CHAPTER 6

DANGEROUS INTERLUDE

W HILE MERCK'S virology operations were developing significant new products and pushing the firm into a strong position
among the U.S. leaders in biologicals, the American economy
was starting its bumpy descent from the prosperity of the American
Century. The years 1965 through 1975 were crucial in this regard, but for
some time it was difficult to perceive what was happening. Government
expenditures for the Vietnam War and for the social welfare "butter" that
President Johnson told the nation it could also afford gave a jump start to
the national economy. Government contracts were available for many
firms. Federal dollars flowed into the science and technology networks,
including those in the medical sciences. But all the while, America's
competitors were rapidly catching up with U.S. firms. Productivity increases in Europe and Asia were running substantially ahead of those in the
United States. The Keynesian jump start also helped launch the Great
Inflation – a development that further weakened the competitive position
of U.S. firms. In 1973 the first oil shock made evident to the general
public what many business executives already knew: the prosperous years
of the American Century were over and the difficult years of intense global
competition had begun.[1]

---

1 Maddison, *Economic Growth in the West*. See also the same author's *Dynamic Forces
in Capitalist Development*. L. Hannah, "Delusions of Durable Dominance or the
Invisible Hand Strikes Back" (draft manuscript, courtesy of the author, 1995).

On the surface, Merck & Co., Inc., appeared to be bucking this trend. Sales increased between 1970 and 1975 by more than 65 percent, reaching $1.26 billion by the latter year. Investors benefited from a two-for-one stock split in 1972, and the price of Merck stock went up by almost 54 percent during the first half of the 1970s.[2] The company was putting more and more money into research and development, which boded well for the long-term future of the enterprise.[3]

But CEO Henry Gadsden was concerned about his company's future in the pharmaceutical industry. In particular, he was anxious about the firm's most important asset, the Merck Sharp & Dohme Research Laboratories. Since the mid-1950s, Merck's strategy had been to bet heavily on MSDRL's ability to develop a steady stream of innovative drugs that would enjoy patent protection and the good sales and relatively high margins that such protection normally ensured. Thus, the company had left vitamin production and distribution when its major products became low-margin commodities. Nor did Merck produce and market generics. Its sales and marketing teams were accustomed to having new blockbuster products on a regular basis and to receiving from the medical community the respect elicited by the Merck name and tradition of innovation.

But as Gadsden knew, the Merck research pipeline was not full of promising drug candidates in the early 1970s. He and his fellow executives decided this was not just one of those temporary flat places that all innovative organizations experience from time to time. The problem was more serious than that. The type of organic chemistry that had been so successful for Merck during the previous four decades was no longer generating the cutting-edge work in medical science. The most promising frontier was now biochemistry, where a new under-

2 Sturchio, ed., *Values and Visions*, pp. 184–5. The sales and stock price figures are in current dollars; the stock prices are yearly averages per share, adjusted for the stock split.

3 Between 1970 and 1975, annual R & D expenditures at Merck jumped from $69 million to $121.9, a 76.6 percent increase (also in current dollars).

standing of disease processes at the molecular level was emerging. While Gadsden was not a scientist, he understood what this development meant for the pharmaceutical industry and especially for Merck. He launched a search for a scientist/science manager capable of quickly positioning Merck at the front edge of the biochemical revolution.

Gadsden and Merck found the leader they wanted at Washington University in St. Louis. Dr. P. Roy Vagelos was director of the university's Division of Biology and Biomedical Sciences and chair of the School of Medicine's Department of Biological Chemistry. His pathbreaking research on the biosynthesis of lipids and the role of cholesterol in the biochemistry of the cell had won him the Enzyme Chemistry Award of the American Chemical Society (1967) and election to the American Academy of Arts and Sciences and the National Academy of Sciences (1972). Persuaded to launch a new career in drug discovery, Vagelos became head of basic research at Merck in 1975 and president of MSDRL the following year.[4]

Vagelos brought to Merck much more than his knowledge of biochemistry and of science management. He introduced in the labora-

---

4 P. Roy Vagelos, M.D., was a native of Rahway, New Jersey, where Merck's headquarters were then located. He received his A.B. from the University of Pennsylvania (1950) and his M.D. from Columbia University (1954). Following his internship and residency at Massachusetts General Hospital in Boston, he spent the years 1956 to 1966 at the National Heart Institute. Appointed as a clinician, he shortly launched a new career as a research scientist in cellular physiology and biochemistry. Inspired by the "terribly exciting" work that enzymologist Earl Stadtman was doing with microbial systems, Vagelos was shortly on the front edge of the research being conducted on microbial enzymes and fatty acid metabolism. He was a codiscoverer of the role of the acyl carrier protein in fatty acid synthesis. In 1966, he left NIH to take over the chairmanship of the Department of Biological Chemistry in the School of Medicine at Washington University in St. Louis, Missouri. Vagelos continued his active research program, working on fatty acid biosynthesis and metabolism, complex lipid synthesis, and finally on the synthesis of cholesterol and the determination of its role in the cell. Before joining Merck in 1975, Vagelos had consulted with MSDRL for several years.

tories a new style of drug discovery. Instead of being dependent upon screening to find new active agents, MSDRL now began to target specific disease processes and to develop drugs that would interfere with those biochemical sequences. The search now focused on chemical entities that would elicit a narrow band of disease-specific responses. While MSDRL continued (to its ultimate advantage) the traditional style of screening, Vagelos made targeted drug discovery the laboratory's central focus. He brought in a new cadre of scientists to implement this program and provide Merck with capabilities in biochemical drug innovation.[5]

1

Vagelos's transformation of MSDRL did not threaten Hilleman's Virus and Cell Biology operation. Nor was the vaccine program endangered when John Horan replaced Henry Gadsden as company president (1975) and then CEO (1976). Horan was committed to MSDRL's role as the prime mover in the firm and was appreciative of what Hilleman's team had accomplished.[6] From Vagelos's perspective, Hilleman was a first-

---

5 See the discussions of this transition in A. Gambardella, "Competitive Advantages from In-House Scientific Research: The U.S. Pharmaceutical Industry in the 1980s," *Research Policy* 21, no. 5 (1992): 391–407. See also F. della Valle and A. Gambardella, " 'Biological' Revolution and Strategies for Innovation in Pharmaceutical Companies," *R&D Management* 23, no. 4 (1993): 287–302; and Gambardella, *Science and Innovation*.

6 Horan was an attorney who had joined Merck's legal department in 1952. He had served as counsel for MSD, the firm's pharmaceutical division, and had subsequently been executive director of research administration for MSDRL (1961–2). After a stint as director of corporate planning, he had returned to MSD, where he was successively executive vice president, general manager, and president. In a talk he gave to the New York Society of Security Analysts (1977), Horan said decisively that Merck intended to remain "one of the leading companies in the world in vaccine research, production, and marketing. With the concept of preventive medicine rapidly gaining broader acceptance, our expertise in this field offers solid growth opportunities." J. J. Horan, "Merck and the Future," May 5, 1977, MA.

rate scientist who was running an organization that was already doing the kind of targeted research that the labs at Rahway were now adopting. So long as Hilleman produced, the new president of the Merck Sharp & Dohme Research Laboratories was not going to tamper with Virus and Cell Biology.

For Hilleman, remaining productive was not a problem, even though he would find it difficult during the 1970s to top the innovations in measles, mumps, and rubella vaccines. While completing the work on the combination vaccine *M-M-R*, he had explored the possibilities of developing a veterinary vaccine for Marek's disease in chickens.[7] As a Montana farm boy, Hilleman had been responsible for the chickens and had learned firsthand about what was then called "range paralysis." The disease was rife among the poultry, where it produced neural tumors and atherosclerosis, killing large numbers of birds. Little was understood about the disease until 1962, when its contagious nature was established. Five years later, using electron microscopy, scientists discovered a herpes-type virus in cells infected with Marek's disease. Shortly afterward, they demonstrated that this particular virus was present in the feather follicles of infected chickens. They had fulfilled Koch's postulates, proving the etiology of the disease.[8] Because it was estimated that as many as 90 percent of the chickens in the United States were infected with the virus, Merck had every reason to support this initiative. For food producers, the potential economic

---

7 Merck had been in the animal health business since the late 1940s, when Max Tishler developed *S.Q.*, a treatment for chicken coccidiosis. Since that time, the company had also introduced two other treatments for coccidiosis (*Nicrazin* and *Amprol*), as well as *Hepzide* (for "blackhead" in turkeys) and *Thibenzole* (an antiparasitic for livestock).

8 M. R. Hilleman, "Marek's Disease Vaccine: Its Implications in Biology and Medicine," *Avian Diseases* 16 (1972): 191–9. Hilleman was particularly intrigued by this project because he had previously done research on the adenoviruses and on SV_{40}, both of which cause neoplastic (that is, tumor-related) changes in animals. At Merck, he had raised the subject of a vaccine as early as 1958. See M. R. Hilleman to M. Tishler and K. Beyer, Nov. 17, 1958, MA.

consequences of a vaccine were extremely significant, particularly after an article appeared pointing out that there was "A Cancer in Every Pot."[9] The U.S. Department of Agriculture routinely condemned chickens with obvious tumors, but as the researchers knew, chickens without such masses could just as likely be infected with the disease. Most cooking methods did not kill the virus.[10]

As Hilleman knew, Marek's disease differed from ordinary viral infections because it was not transmitted by the oral, respiratory, or fecal routes, nor by blood or insect bites. Instead, the infection was spread in the birds' feather follicle cells, by way of infected dander and was not transmitted through the hens' eggs. These two facts made the eradication of Marek's disease a reasonable goal – one that had already been achieved among the chickens Merck was using to prepare *Rubeovax*, its measles virus vaccine. Those chickens were free of Marek's disease as well as avian leukosis, but, of course, they were expensive birds raised and maintained in carefully controlled environments, isolated from viral infection.[11]

---

9 As you might imagine, Merck carefully discussed this subject: M. R. Hilleman to K. Beyer, L. Sarett, and M. Tishler, Feb. 5, 1970; M. R. Hilleman to Fred Bartenstein, Apr. 20, 1970; and M. E. Fletcher to C. Roche, et al., Apr. 21, 1970; all in MA.

10 Although there was no direct proof that the ingestion of diseased chickens could cause cancer in humans, there was no absolute proof to indicate that it could not. Dr. Jack Makari, the head of Makari Research Laboratories in Englewood, New Jersey, warned against the consumption of chicken prepared by most cooking methods, because they failed to kill the Marek's disease virus. Hilleman, "Marek's Disease Vaccine," pp. 191–9. *Pittsburgh Press*, Nov. 8, 1973. J. G. Makari, "Association Between Marek's Herpesvirus and Human Cancer: 1. Detection of Cross-Reacting Antigens Between Chicken Tumors and Human Tumors," *Oncology* 28 (1973): 164–76. But see especially M. R. Hilleman to Those Concerned, Nov. 15, 1973, MA.

11 Memo from M. R. Hilleman to K. Beyer, L. Sarett, and M. Tishler, "Avian Leukosis and Golden Opportunities (Recent Developments and Possibilities for Merck)," Feb. 5, 1970, MA; Hilleman, "Marek's Disease Vaccine," pp. 191–9.

The poultry industry needed a less expensive solution to its problem, and Merck's breakthrough in this instance was a direct result of Hilleman's links to the agricultural and cancer research networks. He and Dr. Benjamin R. Burmester of the USDA's Regional Poultry Research Laboratory (East Lansing, Michigan) shared an interest in avian diseases and cancer. Burmester called Hilleman to say that he had isolated a herpesvirus from turkeys; the virus caused no disease in chickens but it immunized them against Marek's disease. Hilleman was immediately on a plane to Michigan where he obtained the virus.[12]

Even with the virus in hand, it took three years to bring the product to market. One of the problems was to certify that the vaccine would be safe when people ate the chicken. The *Wall Street Journal* voiced concern about this issue, and that too prompted renewed anxiety both at Merck and at the USDA.[13] To eliminate this potential problem, Merck used ten serial passages in isolated chickens to demonstrate continued lack of virulence. Then the vaccine had to be stabilized, prepared for distribution, and subjected to extensive trials.[14]

---

12 B. R. Burmester, "Future Research on the Control of Marek's Disease," *Avian Diseases* 16 (1972): 187–91.

13 M. R. Hilleman to A. Knoppers, Apr. 5, 1971, MA. See also "Government Clears Up Concern About Eating Vaccinated Chickens," *Wall Street Journal*, Apr. 20, 1971. One of the reasons for this concern was that this vaccine worked differently than most others. It established a virus infection that persisted for the bird's lifetime but did not cause clinical disease.

14 R. L. Kilgore, "Prophylactic Efficacy of a Marek's Disease Vaccine in Broiler and Replacement Layer Chickens," *Avian Diseases* 16 (1972): 72–7; in the same issue see also K. A. Honegger, B. L. McMurray, and R. H. Gledhill, "Performance Response of a Leghorn-Type Layer Flock to Turkey Herpesvirus Vaccine," pp. 78–85; J. L. Spencer, A. A. Grunder, A. Robertson, and G. W. Speckmann, "Attenuated Marek's Disease Herpesvirus: Protection Conferred on Strains of Chickens Varying in Genetic Resistance," pp. 94–107; and D. V. Zander, "Commercial Applications of Present Alternatives for Control of Marek's Disease," pp. 179–86.

When these were successful, the U.S. licensed *DEPTAVAC-HVT* in 1971. At first, it was shipped in liquid nitrogen, but this was far too expensive for a poultry industry that could afford to pay only a half cent per dose. Merck answered with a lyophilized, cell-free vaccine that could go through normal shipping channels. [15]

On introduction, the vaccine was an immediate success, but soon Merck confronted intense competition from veterinary vaccine producers. [16] The competition had no development costs to cover and could offer the new product at a significantly lower price. [17] This was the same situation Merck had faced in vitamins and the results were the same. The company discontinued production of the vaccine. This was a setback for Virus and Cell Biology, especially because the department had placed its chickenpox (varicella) vaccine program on hold while working on *DEPTAVAC-HVT*.

As with SV_{40}, there was solace in science. Merck had contributed to the development of the world's first commercial cancer vaccine. There were at this time few leads to the viral etiology of cancer. Researchers working on the viral causes of animal and human cancer were concentrating on two types of retroviruses. Marek's disease was caused by a virus of an entirely different family – a herpesvirus. By demonstrating that infection from an external, transmissible virus

---

15 R. L. Kilgore, "Marek's Disease Vaccine: Prophylactic Efficacy of a Lyophilized Turkey Herpesvirus of Chick Cell-Culture Origin," *Avian Diseases* 17 (1973): 137–41; and the same author's "A Comparison of the Prophylactic Efficacy of Lyophilized and Cell-Associated Turkey Herpesvirus Against Marek's Disease," *Avian Diseases* 18, no. 1 (1974): 45–9.

16 For subsequent indications of efficacy of Merck's vaccine and others see: *Poultry Science* 52 (1973): 836–41, 1450–4, 1482–91, 2009, 2047; 53 (1974): 1533–8, 1946–7. *Progress in Medical Virology* 18 (1974): 178–97. *Avian Diseases* 18, no. 1 (1974): 33–44; 19, no. 2 (1975): 362–5; 22, no. 4 (1978): 583–97.

17 For an indication of the competition that developed see the following: *Avian Diseases* 19, no. 3 (1975): 515–24; 19, no. 4 (1975): 781–90; 21, no. 3 (1977): 440–4; 24, no. 4 (1979): 848–53. M. R. Hilleman, Interview, Nov. 13 and 21, 1991; and M. R. Hilleman, "Notes," MA.

could cause cancer, it followed that prophylactic immunization might be possible. This was an important hypothesis.[18]

There was also a touch of solace in the fact that the Marek's vaccine had an impact on the firm's growth path. Like many other postwar U.S. multinationals, Merck had explored diversification, in part because of fear that the government might limit its future growth in pharmaceuticals with price controls.[19] Unlike many other companies, Merck had remained primarily committed to its core business, but it had diversified.[20] During the 1960s and 1970s, the firm's animal health and vaccine operations guided it toward Hubbard Farms of Walpole, New Hampshire, a business specializing in poultry genetics.[21] In 1974, Merck acquired Hubbard through a stock exchange, and two years later the Hubbard subsidiary acquired SPAFAS, Inc., a producer of specific pathogen free (SPF) fertile eggs and embryos of the sort used extensively in vaccine production. While these diversified enterprises broadened the front across which Merck could innovate, they could hardly compensate for the fact that

---

18 *Medical Tribune*, July 12, 1972. M. R. Hilleman, "Marek's Disease Vaccine," pp. 191–9. See also *Avian Diseases* 20, no. 4 (1976): 676–92; and *Progress in Medical Virology* 22 (1976): 123–51.

19 The events leading up to the passage of the Kefauver-Harris Drug Amendment Act of 1962 had a major impact on Merck's management and especially on the strategic plans of Henry Gadsden, then executive vice president and later CEO. See H. W. Gadsden, "Merck in 1966" (delivered to the Financial Analysts of Philadelphia, Mar. 3, 1966), MA.

20 The acquisitions included Calgon Corporation (1968, water treatment), Baltimore Aircoil Company (1970, water cooling equipment), Kelco Company (1972, alginates and biogums), Pacific Pumping Company (1971, centrifugal pumps), Metalsalts Corporation (1966, specialty chemicals), and Solar Laboratories (1972, lightweight casting systems for fractures). "Acquisitions by Merck & Co., Inc., or a Subsidiary . . . ," Feb. 23, 1972, MA. Sturchio, ed., *Values and Visions*, pp. 28, 30–1, 124.

21 "Hubbard Farms, Inc.," June 28, 1974; A. Viscusi to J. L. Sturchio, Mar. 5, 1990; both in MA. This diversification episode follows rather closely the pattern described in Edith T. Penrose, *The Theory of the Growth of the Firm* (Oxford, 1959).

the company had been unable to recoup its investment in the vaccine for Marek's disease.

2

Nor were the struggles of Hilleman and his colleagues over. The company's influenza vaccines also created more problems in the 1970s than they had in the previous decade. Through the 1960s, Merck had managed to keep its product in a strong position in the national market. This had not been easy because the virus kept changing through either antigenic shift or drift.[22] During the early part of the decade, new strains of the Type B influenza virus had begun to appear in various states around the nation. Although generally less severe than Type A influenza, the new strains of Type B stirred up a great deal of cooperative effort in several corners of the virology network.[23] Scientists and production workers throughout the industry, universities, and various government agencies in America and abroad worked to produce a vaccine of a new composition. Merck played an important role in this international effort and had its version in production even before the DBS had issued its final decisions about the new vaccine.[24]

While clinical tests had by this time established the positive results of influenza vaccination, debate about the procedure contin-

---

22 H. G. Pereira, "Influenza: Antigenic Spectrum," *Progress in Medical Virology* 2 (1969): 46–79; and R. G. Webster and W. G. Laver, "Antigenic Variation in Influenza Virus: Biology and Chemistry," *Progress in Medical Virology* 13 (1971): 271–338. R. F. Betts and R. G. Douglas, "Influenza Virus," in Mandell, Douglas, and Bennett, eds., *Infectious Diseases*, pp. 1306–10.

23 T. D. Y. Chin, W. H. Mosley, J. D. Poland, D. Rush, E. A. Belden, and O. Johnson, "Epidemiologic Studies of Type B Influenza in 1961–1962," *American Journal of Public Health* 53, no. 7 (1963): 1068–74.

24 *Merck Review* 28, no. 1 (1968): 1–7. W. H. Stuart, H. B. Dull, L. H. Newton, J. L. McQueen, and E. R. Schiff, "Evaluation of Monovalent Influenza Vaccine in a Retirement Community During the Epidemic of 1965–1966," *JAMA* 209, no. 2 (1969): 232–8.

ued in both the medical and scientific communities.[25] In epidemics and pandemics, vaccinated persons succumbed to the disease at an incidence 60–75 percent less than the unvaccinated population.[26] But vaccination conferred only temporary immunity (normally for four months), and each time the virus changed, new vaccines had to be developed, approved, and quickly distributed.[27] That was what happened in 1968, when another epidemic occurred in Hong Kong, causing illness in 20 percent of the population. Merck received its first warning in a circular letter from the World Health Organization (Geneva) on August sixteenth. This A_2 virus – aided by modern means of transportation – quickly spread through much of the Asian continent.[28]

The A_2 viral strain rendered the vaccines that had been prepared for that year ineffective. When the DBS received its A_2 seed virus from Japan early in September, the U.S. Surgeon General asked the industry to move swiftly in developing and manufacturing a new vaccine.[29] Of the ten firms licensed to produce influenza vaccines, only

25 R. Batson and R. Sanders, "The Seriologic Response in Children to Asian Influenza-Virus Vaccine," *Pediatrics* 25, no. 6 (1960): 952–5. *American Journal of Public Health* 51, no. 10 (1961): 1596. *JAMA* 208, no. 8 (1969): 1493; 209, no. 12 (1969): 1911; 210, no. 3 (1969): 485–9; 210, no. 10 (1969): 1925; 211, no. 10 (1970): 1672–6; and 212, no. 10 (1970): 1704–6. *New England Journal of Medicine* 270, no. 17 (1964): 870–4; and the commentary in 270, no. 25 (1964): 1366–7; 289, no. 24 (1973): 1309–10. See also *Pediatrics* 41 (1968): 1148–9.

26 *New England Journal of Medicine* 263, no. 19 (1960): 976.

27 See the discussion in *JAMA* 215, no. 7 (1971): 1070, 1073–5.

28 On the A_2 virus see R. Q. Robinson, "Natural History of Influenza Since the Introduction of the A_2 Strain," *Progress in Medical Virology* 6 (1964): 82–110; and W. R. Dowdle, M. T. Coleman, and M. B. Gregg, "Natural History of Influenza Type A in the United States, 1957–1972," *Progress in Medical Virology* 17 (1974): 91–135. Betts and Douglas, "Influenza Virus," p. 1311.

29 M. R. Hilleman, "The Roles of Early Alert and of Adjuvant in the Control of Hong Kong Influenza by Vaccines," *Bulletin of the World Health Organization* 41 (1969): 623–8; *Merck Review* 29, no. 3 (1969): 20–9.

eight were actually active and all of them said they would join the race. At Merck, Hilleman's team of researchers (including some veterans of the 1957 epidemic) went to work at once on the DBS specimens of the new Hong Kong strain. They were under pressure – especially after the Surgeon General announced that high-risk groups should receive both the available polyvalent vaccine and an additional shot of the new Hong Kong vaccine on which Merck and its competitors were just then starting to work.

Merck's target was to make 7,500,000 doses in the time normally allocated to producing one-third that amount. The company created a special task force that dealt with problems ranging from a shortage of embryonated eggs to the need for new equipment. Just over two weeks after the Surgeon General's announcement, the company initiated production of the new killed-virus vaccine and shipped its first 100,000 shots to the West Coast on November 19.[30] By January 20, 1969, Merck had shipped 9,750,000 doses.[31] These shots were used throughout the United States, and even more extensively in South America.[32]

Successful as this effort had been, antigenic change was clearly a significant problem in this wing of the vaccine business.[33] Looking for a way to deal with shift and drift and to make their vaccines generally more effective, Hilleman and his colleagues in the firm and

---

30 *JAMA* 206, no. 10 (1968): 2222. The DBS worked closely with the manufacturers; they simultaneously tested the products for purity and potency in order to accelerate the process. *JAMA* 206, no. 13 (1968): 2836.

31 As in the past, there were problems over allocating the first shots to those most in need of them. *JAMA* 206, no. 10 (1968): 2222; 207, no. 1 (1969): 25.

32 Hilleman, "The Roles of Early Alert and of Adjuvant in the Control of Hong Kong Influenza by Vaccines," pp. 623–8. It was subsequently estimated that the Medicare costs of influenza in 1968–9 were $866,000,000. E. D. Kilbourne, "Influenza," *Preventive Medicine* 3, no. 3 (1974): 461–5.

33 Emergency programs were expensive; at one point during the 1968–9 rush to enhance production capabilities, Merck had as many as one hundred contractors and subcontractors working on tight deadlines to enlarge the firm's facilities.

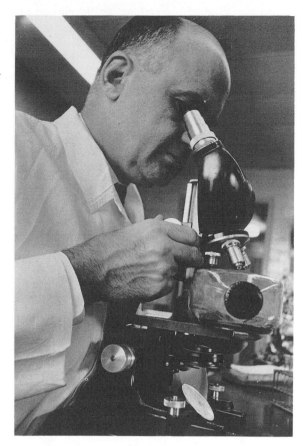

Dr. Maurice R. Hilleman at work in the Merck laboratories.

at the University of Pennsylvania made an interesting discovery during the 1960s. By emulsifying their influenza vaccine in peanut oil, they were able to obtain a higher antibody level of longer duration and broader coverage.[34] Dr. Stokes and his associates confirmed in clinical tests a four to sixteenfold increase in antibody response even when the antigen dose was only at one-quarter strength.[35] Continuing

34 Hilleman, "The Roles of Early Alert and of Adjuvant in the Control of Hong Kong Influenza by Vaccines," pp. 623–8. Adjuvants had earlier been studied in conjunction with polio vaccines. M. R. Hilleman to M. Tishler, June 24, 1958; M. R. Hilleman to M. Tishler and K. Beyer, May 11, 1960; both in MA.

35 Mannide mono-oleate (Arlacel A) was employed as an emulsifier and aluminum monostearate as a stabilizer.

down this line of research, they developed a highly purified aqueous vaccine that, when added to *Adjuvant 65,* greatly enhanced the serologic response to the vaccine. Since the purified vaccine contained less extraneous egg allantoic protein, it was less toxic and less liable to cause allergic reactions.[36] The *Adjuvant 65* formulation also partially overcame the problem of relatively minor viral strain changes.[37] The new preparation, because of its ability to heighten and broaden the antibody response, provided immunity to a greater range of subtypes of the virus.[38]

---

36 The new formula proved to be more durable, as well as more effective. Influenza vaccines in *Adjuvant 65* that were stored at 4° C. for between nine and forty-one months retained their full antigenic potency. See also W. J. McAleer, W. Hurni, E. Wasmuch, and M. R. Hilleman, "High-Resolution Flow-Zonal Centrifuge System," *Biotechnology and Bioengineering* 21, no. 2 (1979): 317–21.

37 Tests in children and the elderly indicated a remarkable enhancement of antibody titers for at least a year. The adjuvant gave Merck a much safer, more effective, and more marketable vaccine. A West Point team of researchers made another improvement when they found that the addition of complex, synthetic polynucleotides (double-stranded RNA) to the vaccine and adjuvant caused a hyperpotentiation of the antibody response. In short, they could magnify even more the immunizing capability of the influenza vaccine and other antigen preparations.

38 A. F. Woodhour, D. P. Metzgar, T. B. Stim, A. A. Tytell, and M. R. Hilleman, "New Metabolizable Immunologic Adjuvant for Human Use: 1. Development and Animal Immune Response," *Proceedings of the Society for Experimental Biology and Medicine* 116 (1964): 516–23. In the same issue see H. M. Peck, A. F. Woodhour, D. P. Metzgar, S. E. McKinney, and M. R. Hilleman, "New Metabolizable Immunologic Adjuvant for Human Use: 2. Short-Term Animal Toxicity Tests," pp. 523–30. J. Stokes, Jr., R. E. Weibel, M. E. Drake, A. F. Woodhour, and M. R. Hilleman, "New Metabolizable Immunologic Adjuvant for Human Use: 3. Efficacy and Toxicity Studies in Man," *New England Journal of Medicine* 271, no. 10 (1964): 479–87. A. F. Woodhour, D. P. Metzgar, G. P. Lampson, R. A. Machlowitz, A. A. Tytell, and M. R. Hilleman, "New Metabolizable Immunologic Adjuvant for Human Use: 4. Development of Highly Purified Influenza Virus Vaccine in Adjuvant 65," *Proceedings of the Society for Experimental Biology and Medicine* 123 (1966): 778–82. A. F. Woodhour, M. R. Hilleman, J. Stokes, Jr., and R. E. Weibel, "Response and Retention of Antibody Following Influenza Virus Vaccine in Adjuvant 65," First International

By the late 1960s, then, Merck appeared to be on the edge of a new era of influenza vaccines. The progress since Sharp & Dohme's first encounter with the vaccine in the 1940s was impressive. Clinical studies indicated that the new formulation of the 1967 vaccine was actually effective against the Hong Kong strain of the virus, stimulating antibody production in more than 50 percent of the recipients.[39] Additional studies conducted in England corroborated this conclusion.[40]

Conference on Vaccines Against Viral and Rickettsial Diseases of Man, *Pan American Health Organization Scientific Publications* 147 (May 1967): 566–9. R. E. Weibel, A. F. Woodhour, J. Stokes, Jr., D. P. Metzgar, and M. R. Hilleman, "New Metabolizable Immunologic Adjuvant for Human Use: 5. Evaluation of Highly Purified Influenza-Virus Vaccine in Adjuvant 65," *New England Journal of Medicine* 276, no. 2 (1967): 78–84. J. Stokes, Jr., R. E. Weibel, A. F. Woodhour, W. J. McAleer, L. A. Potkonski, and M. R. Hilleman, "New Metabolizable Immunologic Adjuvant for Human Use: 9. Large-Scale Trials with Multiple Lots in Different Regimens," *JAMA* 207, no. 11 (1969): 2067–72. See also *Pediatrics* 38, no. 2 (1966): 207–10.

39 A. F. Woodhour, W. J. McAleer, A. Friedman, R. E. Weibel, J. Stokes, Jr., and M. R. Hilleman, "Antibody Response in Man to Hong Kong Influenza Following 1967 Formula Influenza Vaccine in Adjuvant 65," *Proceedings of the Society for Experimental Biology and Medicine* 131 (1969): 501–6.

40 In 1972 the influenza A_2 virus underwent an antigenic drift and caused an epidemic. The virus responsible was substantially different from the A_2 virus that had caused the 1968 epidemic, and the English researchers tried the 1968 vaccine with an adjuvant to see if it would protect against the new viral strain. The results were surprising. In a study in which 83 people received the 1968 A_2 virus in aqueous formulation and 104 received the same vaccine in *Adjuvant 65* formulation, there was a far greater level of antibody titer in the latter group. There was also an excellent broadening of the immunologic response to an antigenically different virus. M. R. Hilleman, A. F. Woodhour, A. Friedman, and R. E. Weibel, "The Safety and Efficacy of Emulsified Peanut Oil Adjuvant 65 When Applied to Influenza Virus Vaccine," International Symposium on Vaccination Against Communicable Diseases, *Symposium Series Immunobiological Standardization* 22 (1973): 107–21. A. F. Woodhour, A. Friedman, R. E. Weibel, and M. R. Hilleman, "Clinical and Laboratory Studies of Improved Adjuvant 65 Influenza Vaccines," *International Symposium on Influenza Vaccines for Men and Horses* 20 (1973): 125–32. See also *New England Journal of Medicine* 289, no. 24 (1973): 1267–71.

But another disappointment followed. Merck's *Adjuvant 65* was licensed in the United Kingdom but not in the United States. The DBS demanded that the preparation be as pure as possible and that it have a well-defined composition. Dr. Karl Pfister and MSDRL's developmental research organization were able to satisfy both of these conditions, but the purified, well-specified formulation no longer worked. Undefined impurities in the original crude material were essential to the adjuvant. Having reached an impasse with the formulation and with the DBS, the company decided not to pursue *Adjuvant 65* any further.[41]

Even more discouraging to Merck was the experience in 1976 with swine influenza. This drama in medical, public health, and political history began at Fort Dix, New Jersey, where a new strain of the influenza virus was discovered. It represented a radical shift from those prevalent at the time and actually resembled the swine influenza virus that Shope had isolated forty-five years before. Even more ominous was the fact that it appeared to be a resurgence of the virus that had caused the lethal 1918–9 pandemic. That possibility quickly produced a sense of panic because one soldier at Fort Dix had died and another five hundred on the base seemed to be infected.[42] The relevant parties in the national vaccine network began to draw together to prepare for this potential crisis.[43] The CDC's Advisory Committee on Immunization Practices (ACIP) concluded that production of a vaccine should start as

---

41 M. R. Hilleman, "Notes," MA. See also *New England Journal of Medicine* 263, no. 19 (1960): 959–62.

42 Richard E. Neustadt and Harvey V. Fineberg, *The Swine Flu Affair: Decision-Making on a Slippery Disease* (Washington, DC, 1978), pp. 5–9. C. M. Cameron to A. A. McLean, Apr. 14, 1976; M. R. Hilleman to R. Hendrickson, May 18, 1976; both in MA.

43 The involved organizations initially included the Centers for Disease Control (CDC), the National Institute of Allergy and Infectious Diseases (NIAID), the Bureau of Biologics (BoB), the U.S. Army, and the New Jersey Department of Health. Ibid., p. 7. Arthur M. Silverstein, *Pure Politics and Impure Science: The Swine Flu Affair* (Baltimore, 1981), pp. 24–8.

soon as possible and that a large-scale public immunization campaign should be initiated.[44]

President Gerald Ford, attempting to cope with an uneasy political present and uncertain future, decided to act more decisively against the swine influenza than he had against inflation. After the Department of Health, Education, and Welfare urged him to take drastic steps to forestall a pandemic, the President convened at the White House (March 24, 1976) a number of the country's top scientists – including its leading virologists – to discuss the issue.[45] Among those present from Merck were Hilleman and Dr. Alan Gray (MSD's director of Biologics). The basis for concern was the discovery of antibodies against swine influenza in a large number of persons throughout the U.S., persons who had been born after the 1918 pandemic. This suggested widespread seeding with the virus. As Hilleman recalls, "It was a stampede to implement a preordained policy!" But neither he nor the other scientists objected to Ford's conclusion that a new National Immunization Program was needed. Congress quickly agreed and allocated the money needed for the new program.[46]

---

44 Ibid., pp. 28–33. *New England Journal of Medicine* 294, no. 19 (1976): 1058–61.

45 J. D. Millar and J. E. Osborn, "Precursors of the Scientific Decision-Making Process Leading to the 1976 National Immunization Campaign," in Osborn, ed., *History, Science, and Politics*, pp. 15–27.

46 A. J. Viseltear, "A Short Political History of the 1976 Swine Influenza Legislation," in Osborn, ed., *History, Science, and Politics*, pp. 29–58. Hilleman later regretted that he had not argued for a compromise position: they should have produced the vaccine, he said, but not implemented mass immunization until there was better evidence that a pandemic would ensue. By June 1976, Hilleman had dug out records he had kept on the first Sharples vaccine made during World War II; examination of that data indicated that the swine flu antibodies found in 1976 were the result of previous immunizations with vaccine containing swine flu. Hilleman advised the U.S. Public Health Service of this conclusion, but the momentum behind the national program was too great to stop the immunizations. M. R. Hilleman, "Notes," MA. See also *New England Journal of Medicine* 295 (1976): 1018.

Never before had the U.S. government initiated such a large-scale public health project. Nor, as it turned out, had one program ever encountered such problems as this one would face.[47] The plan was to have the federal government purchase the vaccine and exercise oversight as it was administered to the U.S. population, largely through public health organizations.[48] Four pharmaceutical companies were involved: Merck; Merrell-National Laboratories; Parke-Davis, and Co.; and Wyeth Laboratories. They were under substantial pressure to have enough doses available to stem the anticipated epidemic.[49]

At Merck, CEO Horan gave overall responsibility for the program to a senior vice president, John L. Huck, who had substantial experience in pharmaceuticals. Horan left little doubt about the importance of the project: "Our products and services meet real needs," he told the stockholders' meeting. "And when our government declares it needs them in the national interest, we will do everything we can to meet that need." Huck had already been attempting to improve the production of biologicals at West Point. It was different, he later said, from pharmaceutical production: "You did it by little recipes, you know, like a person cooks. . . . They were not dealing in precise things as the guys who were doing the chemical work. And that had to change."[50]

Huck had placed an experienced production-line veteran, Frank Ecock, in charge of standardizing and scaling up vaccine manufacturing. This was no small task in an outfit long dominated by an R & D mentality. Ecock made it explicit that the procedures were going

---

47 Dowling, *Fighting Infection*, pp. 201–2; Betts and Douglas, "Influenza Virus," p. 1306. Neustadt and Fineberg, *Swine Flu Affair*, pp. 63–103. Silverstein, *Pure Politics and Impure Science*, pp. 107–42.

48 *American Journal of Public Health* 66, no. 9 (1976): 839–41. Silverstein, *Pure Politics and Impure Science*, pp. 107–15.

49 Dowling, *Fighting Infection*, p. 202.

50 J. L. Huck, Oral History, July 26, 1990, MA.

to change radically: "We were going to make things the same way every day. And we were going to have formulas, and we were going to have procedures." Instead of a laboratory, the facility was going to become "a controlled production environment." He and Hilleman agreed on the principle of standardization, but of course they disagreed about the details. Both men had a good grasp of the fundamentals of organizational combat, and they had some bruising struggles over the production process. Functional concerns about efficiency and control thus prompted Merck to reconsider and change the production operations in Hilleman's highly decentralized vaccine organization.[51] In the end, Ecock and his boss were satisfied that they had improved the operation "at a time when . . . Merck's reputation was . . . on the line."[52]

The government's swine flu program put substantial pressure on the entire organization. Merck's share of the national production schedule was fifty million doses by January 1977. This meant manufacturing in a few months more than five times the amount of influenza vaccine the company normally produced in a year. Instead of 600,000 embryonated eggs a week, Biological Production needed 960,000. The firm added new equipment and new personnel and still had to operate around the clock. Marketing established a liaison with the Centers for Disease Control in Atlanta, which was in charge of distributing the vaccine, and Merck & Co., Inc., was the first to deliver a finished product to the government, sending 11.2 million doses on September 22, 1976.[53]

---

51 Hilleman's organization had a high degree of autonomy vis-à-vis Merck, but within the vaccine operation, authority was centralized.

52 R. Frank Ecock, Interview, Nov. 4, 1991; and M. R. Hilleman, Interview, Nov. 13 and 21, 1991. Hilleman now emphasizes the cooperative nature of this effort more than Ecock does. See M. R. Hilleman, "Notes," MA.

53 R. Frank Ecock, Interview, Nov. 4, 1991. J. L. Huck, Oral History, July 26, 1990, MA.

Unfortunately for Virus and Cell Biology, this performance was quickly pushed out of the headlines by the problems that developed in the entire program. This had already happened once when Merck announced that it was making its vaccine available on a nonprofit, cost-recovery basis. What captured media attention was not this offer, however, but rather a congressional hearing on the liability issue. The pharmaceutical companies and their insurance carriers were understandably concerned about their degree of exposure in circumstances over which they would have no control. As CEO Horan and John Huck explained, Merck was in compliance with government standards on safety and purity but still could be held responsible for the use of the vaccine by third parties without due warning of the possible side effects. The debate dragged on for weeks before Congress passed a law that made the federal government responsible for the outcome of immunization in this instance.[54]

Then came the program's second major crisis. As events at this time clearly indicated, the manufacturers' concerns about liability had been justified. The inoculation program had been going for just two weeks when three elderly people in a Pittsburgh clinic died shortly after receiving the vaccine. Pittsburgh discontinued its inoculation program and eight states followed. Investigations began and concern increased when deaths among the elderly in other states were linked to the vaccine. In the field trials, the vaccine had been effective, with no serious clinical reactions. So convincing was this evi-

---

54 Given the decision in *Reyes v. Wyeth* (1974), the manufacturers had every reason to be worried about liability. In that case, the company had been held liable for damages when an infant contracted polio after receiving Wyeth's Sabin live-virus vaccine. The company had included warnings in printed form, but the court held that the warning was inadequate. For an excellent discussion of the liability issue see E. W. Kitch and E. A. Mortimer, Jr., "American Law, Preventive Vaccine Programs, and the National Vaccine Compensation Program," in Plotkin and Mortimer, eds., *Vaccines*, pp. 933–57. On the 1976 situation, see Neustadt and Fineberg, *The Swine Flu Affair*, pp. 48–62.

dence that the national director of the immunization program, Dr. Delano Meriweather, announced that there was no connection between the vaccine and these deaths. The deaths, he said, could be traced to complications of other illnesses.

The vaccine appeared to have been vindicated – but not for long. Approximately forty-five million people received the vaccine and in the span of three months it was linked to a significant rise in the occurrence of Guillain-Barre Syndrome (GBS), a neuromuscular disease. GBS is a relatively rare disease that resulted in a gradual, but usually temporary, paralysis and had a mortality rate of 5 percent. Since the preliminary statistics suggested that there were higher rates of GBS among vaccinees, the government suspended the immunization program as a precautionary measure until a full investigation could be completed.[55] In subsequent decades influenza vaccine would be used extensively (with fifteen to eighteen million shots administered annually by the early 1980s), without problems involving Guillain-Barre Syndrome.[56] But in 1976, the resulting controversy killed the national program.

Then, as a final blow to this experiment in national preventive medicine, the anticipated epidemic did not materialize in the winter of

---

55 The figures resulting from the subsequent studies have been contested, but see Silverstein, *Pure Politics and Impure Science*, pp. 120–3 for a careful examination of the evidence. The total number of "excess cases" was not large, but the linkage was "statistically significant." A. D. Langmuir, D. J. Bregman, L. T. Kurland, N. Nathanson, and M. Victor, "An Epidemiologic and Clinical Evaluation of Guillain-Barre Syndrome Reported in Association with the Administration of Swine Influenza Vaccines," *American Journal of Epidemiology* 119, no. 6 (1984): 841–79.

For a different conclusion see M. R. Hilleman, "Notes," MA. See also *American Journal of Public Health* 69, no. 3 (1979): 219–21. And *Lancet* (Jan. 29, 1977): 253–4.

56 *Merck Review* 38, no. 1 (1977): 26–33; Dowling, *Fighting Infection*, p. 202; Betts and Douglas, "Influenza Virus," pp. 1320–1.

1976–7. As Hilleman observed, the swine influenza at Fort Dix appeared to be a zoonosis that "just didn't make the grade in man."[57] In the following years, the science related to the influenza vaccines continued to evolve.[58] As it did, Merck's killed-virus vaccine lost market share to so-called split or subunit influenza vaccines.[59] Although less immunogenic than the whole-virus product, they were less toxic and – not to be ignored by a business – were preferred by pediatricians.[60]

57 M. R. Hilleman, "Serologic Responses to Split and Whole Swine Influenza Virus Vaccines in Light of the Next Influenza Pandemic," *Journal of Infectious Diseases* 136, supp. (1977): S683–5. See also *New England Journal of Medicine* 295, no. 14 (1976): 785–6; and Joseph A. Bellanti and Vijaya L. Melnick, eds., *Symposium on Public Concerns of Immunization* (Baltimore, 1979), which prints proceedings from a conference prompted by the abortive Swine Flu program.

58 One development involved an effective chemotherapeutic agent, amantadine, manufactured by Du Pont. In America, this product had been licensed for general use in 1966 as a prophylactic tool against the influenza A_2 virus. By 1976, it had received approval as a therapeutic agent and for application against all Type A viruses. It appears not to have become popular in this country in part because of side effects in some recipients. Meanwhile, increasing the antigenic mass in the vaccines had improved the antibody response. This was particularly efficacious for the elderly. Significant progress has also been made in measuring the quantity of virus in a vaccine through immunodiffusion. Betts and Douglas, "Influenza Virus," pp. 1306, 1320. See also *New England Journal of Medicine* 298, no. 11 (1978): 621–2. A. S. Beare, "Live Viruses for Immunization Against Influenza," *Progress in Medical Virology* 20 (1975): 49–83. And *Lancet* (May 13, 1972): 1039–40.

59 *JAMA* 230, no. 6 (1974): 863–6. *Virology* 69 (1976): 511–22. *New England Journal of Medicine* 296, no. 10 (1977): 567–8.

60 P. A. Gross, G. V. Quinnan, P. F. Gaerlan, C. R. Denning, A. Davis, M. Lazicki, and M. Bernius, "Potential for Single High-Dose Influenza Immunization in Unprimed Children," *Pediatrics* 70, no. 6 (1982): 982–6. See also *Pediatrics* 52, no. 3 (1973): 416–19; and 69, no. 4 (1982): 404–8. *American Journal of Public Health* 69, no. 12 (1979): 1247–51. But compare *New England Journal of Medicine* 296, no. 25 (1977): 1477–8. Hilleman's position was that the subunit vaccines would not deal effectively with the next pandemic and that Merck should continue with the whole-virus line. M. R. Hilleman, "Notes," MA.

Beset by questions of liability, by the inevitable problems of high-pressure efforts to develop new vaccines, and by the loss of market share, Merck abandoned the influenza vaccine business to its small number of active competitors a few years later.[61]

3

These events of the 1970s and the economic problems the entire vaccine industry were encountering prompted Merck to reconsider its investment in biologicals. "Is the Human Vaccines business a good business to be in?" the 1979 *Vaccine Study* asked. By that time, Vagelos had the Merck Sharp & Dohme Research Laboratories set securely on a new and promising course. In 1978, the firm had rolled out three new drugs in the American market: *Timoptic*, for the treatment of glaucoma; *Clinoril*, a nonsteroidal, anti-inflammatory for relief of arthritis; and *Mefoxin*, an injectible antibiotic.[62] Equally important were the promising drug candidates in the MSDRL pipeline. All of these products – current and future – were assured of patent protection in the United States and many of them would find significant markets abroad.[63] The success in pharmaceuticals left the biological operations vulnerable to the kind of intrafirm struggle over resources that constantly shapes and reshapes corporate capabilities.[64]

The 1979 *Vaccine Study* acknowledged the success Merck had achieved in vaccines in the past two decades. Under Hilleman's leadership, the company had become the largest producer of human vaccines in the world, and it had done so with fewer products than many of its competitors. Given the condition Merck's biological operation had

---

61 Press release, Oct. 13, 1982, MA.

62 Merck & Co., Inc., *1978 Annual Report*, MA.

63 The company had already launched *Dolobid*, a new prescription analgesic, in the United Kingdom, Portugal, and Nigeria, while the U.S. clinical studies were being completed. Ibid.

64 L. Galambos, "The Authority and Responsibility of the Chief Executive Officer: Shifting Patterns in Large U.S. Enterprises in the Twentieth Century," *Industrial and Corporate Change* 4, no. 1 (1995): 190–1.

been in during the mid-1950s, this was a commendable record of growth and innovation in a line of products that had continued to be profitable through the past ten years.[65]

But the profits were a growing concern, and the basic thrust of the study was negative about the industry and about Merck's future in vaccines. The industry was "ailing," and not just in the United States: "No company currently not in the vaccines business would (logically) choose to get in." The total world market was small — around the $200,000,000 range — and about half of that was in the United States. In America and overseas, margins were tight, with many old products selling as commodities. As a result, there were only about a dozen competitors of any significance left among the capitalist industrial nations, and in recent years several of the largest vaccine producers in the United States had left the business. Pfizer, Lilly, Dow, and Richardson-Merrell had given up. That left Lederle, Parke-Davis, Wyeth, and Connaught as the major competitors in the U.S. market.

Overseas markets were difficult for Merck Sharp & Dohme International (MSDI) to crack. A number of the European companies were looked on by their governments as "national institutions": Pasteur and Mérieux, both in France, and Behringwerke in Germany were the Big Three. Mérieux, which produced a complete line of human vaccines, had annual sales in the $20 to $30 million range, two-thirds of them in France. Pasteur was government owned. While its annual sales of human vaccines were only about $15 million, it had a research budget of $40 million. Behringwerke, part of Hoechst, marketed almost exclusively in Germany and had annual sales less than $20 million. Although Merck (with human vaccine sales of $65.6 million in 1978) was much larger than any of these firms, they had the support of their national governments, as did Sclavo in Italy, RIT in Belgium and Holland, and Burroughs-Welcome and Glaxo in the United King-

---

65 This and all subsequent references to the vaccine study refer to H. Lipmanowicz, *Vaccine Study – 1979* (Aug. 1979), MA.

Dr. Hilleman's daughter, Jeryl Lynn, provides moral support as her son is vaccinated with M-M-R II, containing mumps vaccine made from the original Jeryl Lynn strain of virus.

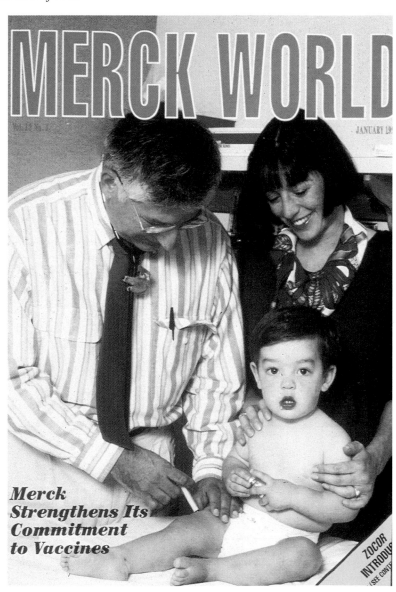

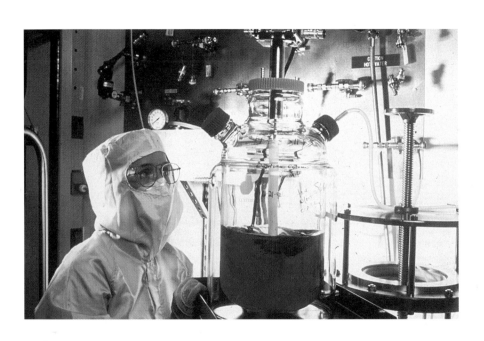

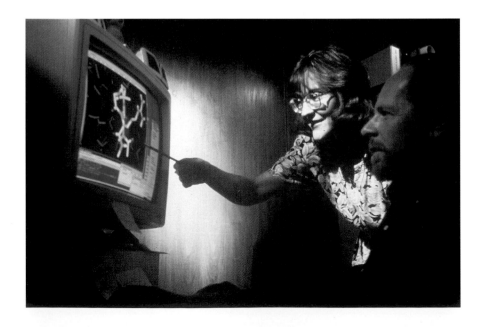

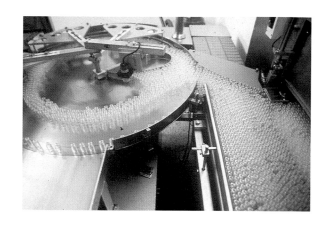

Left, top. *Engineer Julie Camburn enters data during the manufacturing process for Merck's hepatitis A vaccine,* Vaqta.

Bottom. *Dr. Dennis Underwood and Dr. Kristine Prendergast of the Merck Research Laboratories use computer modeling in their discussion of future vaccines.*

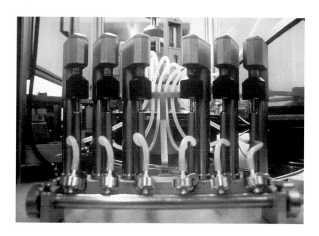

Right, top. *Clean glassware is transferred mechanically in Merck's sterile filling and packaging operations.*

Center. *Vials of Recombivax HB are filled, sealed, and quality tested.*

Bottom. *Vials of vaccine being weighed individually at Merck.*

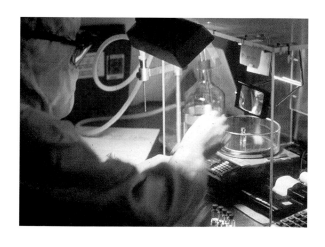

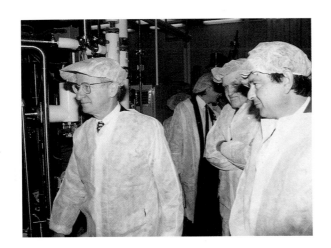

R. Gordon Douglas, Jr., M.D., President of Merck Vaccines, tours the recombinant DNA vaccine facility Merck built for the Peoples Republic of China. (1993)

Bottom. *Dedication ceremony (1993) in China for the opening of the recombinant DNA vaccine production plant.*

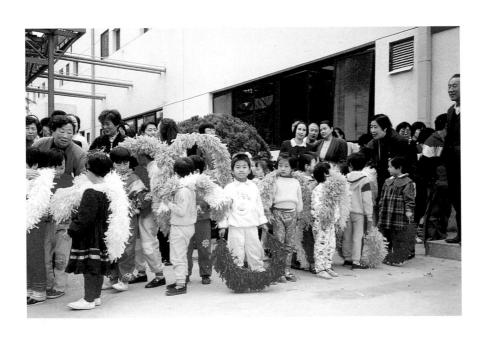

dom. As a result, MSDI at that time was making no vaccine sales in France, Germany, Britain, Italy, or Spain.

In its own home market, Merck did not have the kind of positive relationship with its government that the European competitors had with theirs. Seeking lower prices, the government had encouraged the development of "generic vaccine houses" that did not have research and development costs and could operate with smaller profit margins.[66] Merck had avoided price increases when it was the sole supplier of vaccines used in statewide or nationwide immunization programs.[67] In the important pediatrics market, the firm had a large contract with the Centers for Disease Control at prices that yielded little profit. While prices remained relatively stable, the costs in the vaccine operations had increased sharply, especially in research.[68] Merck's return on vaccine investments had fallen off since its 1970 peak, reaching 2.9 percent during the disastrous swine flu episode of 1976.

While R & D costs were increasing, Virus and Cell Biology had hit a relatively flat phase of innovation in the 1970s. As late as 1975, the vaccine organization had predicted that it would have thirteen new human and two new animal vaccines licensed by 1980. Only two were forthcoming, however, and one of these had insignificant sales.[69] The 1979 study forcefully contended that without a high rate of sustained innovation, the vaccine business could not be conducted on a profitable basis: "In the end, the answer to the question 'is it worth it' can only come from research."

While Merck's executives were pondering the company's future in biologicals, the federal government was also beginning to express

---

66 See, for instance, Chapter 5.

67 This had also been the case in the abortive swine flu immunization program.

68 This trend was also evident in pharmaceutical research in general. J. A. DiMasi, R. W. Hansen, H. G. Grabowski, and L. Lasagna, "Cost of Innovation in the Pharmaceutical Industry," *Journal of Health Economics* 10 (1991): 107–42.

69 We cover these two vaccines, *Meningovax A/C* and *Pneumovax*, in Chapter 7.

concern about the declining rate of innovation in vaccines. Paradox notwithstanding, the same government that had helped create economic and legal conditions that hampered innovation in this wing of the private sector now became worried about what was *not* happening. The National Institute of Allergy and Infectious Diseases (NIAID, part of the National Institutes of Health) proposed that the government set up a program to accelerate development of new vaccines. The Department of Health and Human Services, which had a Steering Committee for Development of a Health Research Strategy, would conduct the program. The Steering Committee recommended NIAID's proposal to Health and Human Services, which of course organized a meeting and launched a multinetwork, nonprofit/private-sector/public, three-pronged study of the problem. One prong involved "establishing priorities" for "diseases of importance in the United States." Another set priorities for "diseases of importance in developing countries." The third looked at the vital area of "public-private sector relations in vaccine innovation." Maurice R. Hilleman carried Merck's flag as a participant in all three of the studies, which, like most such multinetwork ventures, would take several years to produce results.[70]

For the present, Hilleman and his coworkers had much more pressing concerns at home, in Rahway, New Jersey. Within Merck, the *Vaccine Study – 1979* was a serious challenge to the biological operations. Particularly telling were the figures on the increases in research expenditures and assets and the accompanying decline in return on investment. Why, the study asked, did Merck's competitors remain in this "ailing" industry? "The reasons are mostly *NOT* of the 'rational, strictly business' type. The major one for many is political." Then, too, "inertia prevails." It did not take too much imagination to conclude

---

70 Institute of Medicine, Committee on Issues and Priorities for New Vaccine Development, *New Vaccine Development: Establishing Priorities*, vol. 1, *Diseases of Importance in the United States*; vol. 2, *Diseases of Importance in Developing Countries*; and Institute of Medicine, Division of Health Promotion and Disease Prevention, *Vaccine Supply and Innovation* (all three published Washington, DC, 1985).

that some "rational, strictly business" executives at Merck's Rahway headquarters might see the advantages in overcoming inertia and shifting the vaccine resources to a more promising part of the company.[71] Ominously, the report concluded, the basic conditions that had prevailed in the 1970s were unlikely to change during the next few years.

---

71 The study said that Merck's problem was "not how to get out of the vaccine business but how to manage its vaccine business so that it can be returned to a healthy level of growth and profitability." The author made a number of positive proposals for improving the vaccine operations. But throughout, the report echoed, "Must we pull out of the vaccine business?"

CHAPTER 7

TRANSFORMING BACTERIOLOGY:
A SECOND PHASE

T HE LEADER of the Merck Sharp & Dohme Research Laboratories responded forcefully to the negative conclusions of the
Vaccine Study – 1979. P. Roy Vagelos was trained as a physi-
cian, and although he had spent most of his career in science, he had never
abandoned the values of medical practice. Those values were reflected in
his response to the vaccine report, and the reasoning was straightforward:
Merck's primary mission was to develop effective treatments for human
and animal diseases. The best treatment for any disease was prevention.
Vaccines prevented disease and Hilleman's organization had for some years
now been the most successful in the nation in developing new and important vaccines. They had promising innovations in the pipeline. Without
challenging the economic data indicating that Merck should follow several
of its former competitors and leave the vaccine business, Vagelos argued
strongly that Merck should stay the course. CEO Horan decided to go
along with Vagelos – and Hilleman.[1]

1

There was evidence on both sides of this issue in the work Virus and
Cell Biology had been doing recently in developing vaccines for bacterial infections. Hilleman, who had spent his entire adult life working
with viruses, had not been eager to transfer his talents and those of his

---

1 Interviews with P. Roy Vagelos, Jan. 12 and 23, 1995.

research team into bacteriology. "The point was," he later recalled, "that if you're doing virology and you have an overwhelming amount of work to do, you don't take on something else." Max Tishler was persistent, however, and after the great push to complete the measles, mumps, and rubella vaccines was over, Virus and Cell Biology began to explore bacterial vaccines.[2]

During this second phase of innovation, the first two vaccines approved by the government were clinical success stories – but only one of them had substantial market potential. The first to be licensed, *Meningovax-C*, prevented meningitis, an infection that was one of those most feared by the public, although it was by no means the most deadly. It was feared in part because it often occurred in closed populations and in part because it could cause death so quickly, in a matter of hours in some cases. As one commentator in the 1970s observed: "Except, perhaps, for rabies and smallpox, there is almost no other infectious disease which tends to upset and to paralyze so many people and to create such mass hysteria."[3]

Prior to the development of effective vaccines, treatment had for some years consisted of serum antitoxins; later, physicians had used serum in combination with antibiotics. Mulford had, for many years, produced a serum antitoxin for meningococcal disease.[4] With serum treatments alone – before the development of sulfonamides and penicillin – mortality had been about 50 percent.[5] The sulfa drugs and penicillin had significantly reduced that figure, but by the 1960s doctors were encountering meningococci so resistant to sulfonamides that they

---

2 M. R. Hilleman, Interview, Nov. 13 and 21, 1991.

3 H. A. Feldman, "Some Recollections of the Meningococcal Diseases," *JAMA* 220, no. 8 (1972): 1107–12. See also D. H. Smith, D. L. Ingram, A. L. Smith, F. Gilles, and M. J. Bresnan, "Bacterial Meningitis: Diagnosis and Treatment," *Pediatrics* 52, no. 4 (1973): 586–600.

4 See Chapter 2.

5 But as late as 1971, the mortality rate among children under two years old was above 30 percent. *JAMA* 216, no. 9 (1971): 1424.

could be eliminated neither from the carriers nor the patients with this disease. An outbreak of the disease among military recruits in 1963 prompted the Armed Forces Epidemiological Board to launch a new search for vaccines.[6]

In 1969, a team at Walter Reed led by E. C. Gotschlich, I. Goldschneider, and M. S. Artenstein developed highly purified vaccines for two forms of the meningococci, groups A and C.[7] These vaccines used high-molecular-weight polysaccharide antigens from the capsules of meningococci. The Gotschlich-Goldschneider-Artenstein group administered their vaccine for group C to 13,763 Army recruits and discovered that it was 87 percent effective. It reduced the carrier state to a significant degree and produced no systemic adverse reactions.[8] The new vaccine would provide protection for groups in closed settings like the military, schools, and prisons.[9]

---

6 N. A. Vedros, D. H. Hunter, and J. H. Rust, Jr., "Studies on Immunity in Meningococcal Meningitis," *Military Medicine* 131, no. 11 (1966): 1413–17. Feldman, "Some Recollections," pp. 1107–12. M. A. Apicella, "Neisseria Meningitidis," in Mandell, Douglas, and Bennett, eds., *Infectious Diseases*, pp. 1600–13. Theodore E. Woodward, *The Armed Forces Epidemiological Board: Its First Fifty Years* (Falls Church, VA, 1990), pp. 83, 92, 340–4. On sulfa-resistant organisms see also *New England Journal of Medicine* 287, no. 1 (1972): 5–9.

7 Type A was rare in the United States, but was the most common form of the disease elsewhere in the world (and especially in Africa). Type A outbreaks tended to come in ten- to twelve-year cycles. In 1964, most of the cases in the U.S. Army were a product of group B, but by 1970, group C accounted for 96 percent of the disease. *Lancet* (Mar. 18, 1972): 625. Vedros, Hunter, and Rust, "Studies on Immunity in Meningococcal Meningitis," p. 1413.

8 W. E. Bell and D. L. Silber, "Meningococcal Meningitis: Past and Present Concepts," *Military Medicine* 136, no. 7 (1971): 601–11. The vaccines were also tested in children aged seven months to ten years. *JAMA* 216, no. 9 (1971): 1419–20.

9 M. S. Artenstein, R. Gold, P. E. Winter, and C. D. Smith, "Immunoprophylaxis of Meningococcal Infection," *Military Medicine* 139, no. 2 (1974): 91–5. Later, they developed a vaccine against group A, the more common form among populations that are not closed. *JAMA* 220, no. 12 (1972): 1548.

After representatives from the U.S. Army discussed this situation with Max Tishler, he persuaded Hilleman to venture into the chemistry of polysaccharides. The company's Virus and Cell Biology operation developed and Merck manufactured for the armed services a capsular, group C vaccine that the Army and Navy gave to all of their recruits on induction. By 1974, the Merck product had been used with more than 350,000 military personnel, with excellent results.[10] Merck also developed a vaccine for group A and used both vaccines in extensive clinical trials[11] with civilian and military populations.[12]

---

10 The initial military contract was for 400,000 doses of group C and 100,000 doses of group A vaccine. Subsequent contracts into 1975 were for almost two million doses of group C vaccine. *Meningovax* Backgrounder, Jan. 13, 1975, MA.

11 The organization of the Finnish clinical trials was typical of the manner in which programs developed in these networks. Hilleman contacted the public health laboratory in Finland, which arranged for the tests in that country; because public health did not have sufficient funds to support the tests, Merck supplied some of the money, as did the National Institute of Allergy and Infectious Diseases and the Sigrid Juselius Foundation. M. R. Hilleman to J. Mantovaara, Oct. 17, 1974, MA. P. H. Mäkelä, H. Käyhty, P. Weckström, A. Sivonen, and O. Renkonen, "Effect of Group-A Meningococcal Vaccine in Army Recruits in Finland," *Lancet* (Nov. 8, 1975): 883–6.

12 Mäkelä, Käyhty, Weckström, Sivonen, and Renkonen, "Effects of Group-A Meningococcal Vaccine in Army Recruits in Finland," pp. 883–6. R. E. Weibel, V. M. Villarejos, P. P. Vella, A. F. Woodhour, A. A. McLean, and M. R. Hilleman, "Clinical Laboratory Investigations of Monovalent and Combined Meningococcal Polysaccharide Vaccines, Groups A and C," *Proceedings of the Society for Experimental Biology and Medicine* 153 (1976): 436-40. Dr. P. Helena Mäkelä of the Central Public Health Laboratory and Dr. Osvald Pettay of the University Central Hospital conducted the clinical tests in Finland, which had experienced a meningitis epidemic since early 1973. Children as well as military personnel took part in the tests. See also *JAMA* 230, no. 10 (1974): 1458; 231, no. 3 (1975): 234.

Hilleman completed the arrangements for the Finnish clinical trials – for which Merck donated the vaccines – without contacting Merck Sharp & Dohme's office in Finland. This brought an anguished response from the MSD

Based on these results, the company applied for a license for *Meningovax-C*.[13]

Both the U.S. government and Merck were under substantial pressure at this time to provide vaccines to those parts of the world experiencing epidemics – and to those Americans who worked or traveled there. Nevertheless, the Bureau of Biologics delayed because of concern about the evidence indicating that in rabbit tests the Merck product frequently caused fevers. Since the clinical tests produced no supporting data, however, the Food and Drug Administration finally licensed *Meningovax-C* (April 1974) for use in epidemics.[14] This gave Merck permission to export the new product, first to Brazil, which was suffering a serious public health problem with meningitis.[15] So acute was the pressure to provide supplies for that Latin American country that Merck's production line was initially strained beyond its capacity. Demand in the United States was intense as well, both for those traveling to Latin America and for those in communities experiencing

---

office, which thought a public announcement should have been made. Hilleman, who was not an easy man to bend toward corporate concerns, replied: "One does not conduct public relations with research. This is a high level ethical thing and it has nothing to do with the donation of vaccine." M. R. Hilleman to J. Mantovaara, Oct. 17, 1974, MA.

13 *JAMA* 228, no. 5 (1974): 557–8; also 229, no. 10 (1974): 1287. Press release, Apr. 4, 1974, MA.

14 Press release, Apr. 4, 1974, MA. See also *JAMA* 235, no. 1 (1976): 14. By 1976, Merrell-National Laboratories, as well as Merck, was licensed to produce both the C and A vaccines. On pyrogenicity see M. R. Hilleman, Interview, Nov. 13 and 21, 1991. On the demand from Brazil see F. Rodriguez to J. R. Piccin, Oct. 25, 1974, MA.

15 On the pressure to supply Brazil see J. Stuart to F. Rodriguez, Nov. 22 and 25, 1974. Also, Piccin to de Santis/Vouto, Nov. 25, 1974. The French firm Institut Mérieux was also supplying both A and C vaccines and was under similar pressure; see "Merieux Denies Delay in the Delivery of Vaccines," Nov. 7, 1974. All in MA. See also *New York Times*, May 11, 1975; and *Time*, Sept. 9, 1974.

outbreaks.[16] It was the year's end before these problems were behind Merck, which by that time had supplied 3,000,000 doses to Brazil alone.[17]

Although Hilleman and his group subsequently improved their vaccines' purity and reduced their pyrogenicity; although the government licensed their A and combined (A and C) vaccines; although meningitis vaccines were used extensively in Africa; although subsequent tests indicated that the vaccines could be effective in the most vulnerable age group, very young children – despite all of this, *Meningovax* was not a profitable innovation capable of winning over those within Merck who were sceptical about the vaccine business.[18] Like the influenza vaccine, *Meningovax* was only needed periodically;

---

16 The Meningococcal Disease Surveillance Group, "Meningococcal Disease," *JAMA* 235, no. 3 (1976): 261–5. JWS to JEF, Aug. 9, 1974. A. Weymouth to A. J. Boyd, Aug. 27, 1974. J. Stuart to Dr. Friedrich, Oct. 9, 1974. R. C. Bostwick to J. E. Fletcher, et al., with enclosures, Oct. 15, 1974. F. Rodriguez to A. Monserrat, Oct. 17, 1974. A. C. True to Dear Doctor, Jan. 27, 1975. All in MA. One of the domestic outbreaks was in Trenton, N.J. *Philadelphia Inquirer*, Nov. 22 and 24, 1974. See also R. C. Bostwick to J. E. Fletcher, et al., Nov. 22, 1974; and R. C. Bostwick to M. R. Hilleman, Dec. 5, 1974; both in MA.

17 R. Bostwick to J. W. Stuart and S. Weymouth, Sept. 4, 1974; R. Bostwick to Hilleman, Dec. 5, 1974; *Medical World News*, Aug. 23, and Oct. 25, 1974; all in MA. R. Frank Ecock, Interview, Nov. 4, 1991.

18 M. R. Hilleman, "Notes," MA. On African immunization campaigns see World Health Organization, Study Group on Cerebrospinal Meningitis Control, "Cerebrospinal Meningitis Control," *World Health Organization Technical Report Series* 588 (1976): 5–29; *New York Times*, July 25, 1974; *Medical Week*, Nov. 8, 1974; *JAMA* 236, no. 5 (1976): 459–61; *Lancet* (July 11, 1981): 80–2, and *Lancet* (Aug. 7, 1981): 315–17. By 1976 the following groups had been identified: A, B, C, D, X, Y, Z, Z', and W135. On Merck's problems supplying Zambia with *Meningovax* see R. A. Johnson to L. F. Fayet, with attachments, Nov. 24, 1975, MA. Merck had destroyed the first two batches of vaccine allocated to Zambia because they had not met the standards of the company's quality control operations. This had caused problems with the customer, the Ministry of Health. On vaccinating young children see *JAMA* 238, no. 17 (1977): 1804; and *Pediatrics* 60, no. 5 (1977): 673–80.

---

and the periods were further apart and the endangered populations in Merck's primary market, the United States, far less extensive than was the case with flu.[19] There were several competitors in the market within a few years; that too influenced the potential return on the firm's investment.[20] In the aftermath of the 1979 vaccine study, Merck tightened its belt and left the market for meningitis vaccines.[21]

2

More promising as a commercial venture was the work Virus and Cell Biology had started on a pneumonia vaccine. Like so many of these research projects, this one began through personal ties, in this case between Hilleman and Dr. Robert Austrian of the University of Pennsylvania School of Medicine. Austrian had for years battled the ruling forces in the medical and bacteriological networks. He contended that chemotherapy against pneumococcal disease was inadequate during the first five days of infection. Because many patients died during those five days, Austrian had persisted in advocating preventive immunization.[22]

The debate over chemotherapy versus immunization – which had been going on in one form or another for decades – was important: during the 1970s, pneumonia was the fifth leading cause of death in

---

19 See the discussion in *JAMA* 243, no. 24 (1980): 2525-6; also *Lancet* (Dec. 2, 1978): 1185–6; *New England Journal of Medicine* 308, no. 23 (1983): 1421.

20 In addition to Merrell, Squibb and Connaught Laboratories produced meningitis vaccines. *Military Medicine* 139, no. 2 (1974): 91; and 150, no. 10 (1985): 529.

21 M. R. Hilleman, "Notes," MA; and M. R. Hilleman, Interview, Nov. 13 and 21, 1991.

22 Robert Austrian, *Life with the Pneumococcus: Notes from the Bedside, Laboratory, and Library* (Philadelphia, 1985). M. R. Hilleman, "Notes," MA. There was also evidence of resistant forms of pneumococcus. See, for instance, W. Schaffner, W. M. Schreiber, and M. G. Koenig, "Fatal Pneumonia Due to a Tetracycline-Resistant Pneumococcus," *New England Journal of Medicine* 274, no. 8 (1966): 451–2.

---

the United States, and in 1976 alone, about 753,000 cases required hospitalization. In normal circumstances, pneumococci live in the throats of about half of all people without causing disease. But pathology ensues when the bacteria invade the lung (pneumonia), the middle ear (otitis media), the blood (bacteremia), and the brain (meningitis).[23] Pneumonia takes a heavy toll in deaths, suffering, and healthcare costs. In addition to the elderly population, people with chronic heart, lung, kidney, and metabolic diseases and diabetes are at high risk.[24]

The efforts to treat or prevent the disease have a long and complex history, one phase of which – as we saw in Chapter 2 – involved the serum treatments that the Mulford Company developed in the early 1900s. In the 1920s and 1930s, improvements in the typing of pneumococci and in the concentration and purification of serums resulted in widespread use of serum treatment. The process of determining the type of the infecting pneumococcus was still laborious, but a study in the early 1940s indicated that less than 15 percent of the patients treated in this manner died.[25]

After Sharp & Dohme acquired Mulford in 1929, S & D continued to produce a concentrated pneumococcus antibody globulin solution. This product consisted of the active antibodies from antipneumococcic serum types 1 and 2, combined in a salt solution. At that time, these two types were responsible for most cases of the disease.[26] Using either mice or S & D's rabbit sera tests, physicians could determine the specific type of pneumonia they were treating and

---

23 P. Smit, D. Oberholzer, S. Hayden-Smith, H. J. Koornhof, and M. R. Hilleman, "Protective Efficacy of Pneumococcal Polysaccharide Vaccines," *JAMA* 238, no. 24 (1977): 2613–16. See also *New England Journal of Medicine* 274, no. 23 (1966): 1285–9.

24 M. A. Mufson, "Streptococcus Pneumoniae," in Mandell, Douglas, and Bennett, eds., *Infectious Diseases*, p. 1543.

25 Dowling, *Fighting Infection*, pp. 47–9.

26 *S & D Extract* 4, no. 2 (1931), MA.

prescribe the appropriate serum therapy.[27] The company also produced at the Glenolden laboratories both bacterins (killed bacteria in a buffered salt solution) and serobacterins (an antibody-antigen combination) for the treatment of pneumonia.[28] Then, as now, treatment was complicated by the fact that there are at least eighty-five different serologic types of the pneumococci bacteria.[29]

These complications disappeared, along with serum treatment, after the introduction of sulfapyridine in 1939 and penicillin in the 1940s. So effective did these new drugs appear to be that neither serums nor vaccines were in demand, even though considerable progress had been made in developing vaccines. Building on the pioneering research of Michael Heidelberger and Oswald Avery, Colin MacLeod had used the polysaccharide capsule from the bacterium to develop a

---

27 *S & D Abstract* 9, no. 3 (1937): 3–15, MA. By mixing bacteria from the patient with specific pneumococcus antisera, it was possible to determine which serotype was causing the infection and hence which specific serum should be used for treatment. The indication for a match in type was by microscopic observation for swelling of the pneumococcus capsule (Quellung Reaction). M. R. Hilleman, "Notes," MA. Austrian, *Life with the Pneumococcus*, pp. 37–49. See also H. F. Dowling, "Diphtheria as a Model: Introduction of Serums and Vaccines for Scarlet Fever and Pneumococcal Pneumonia," *JAMA* 226, no. 5 (1973): 550–3.

28 *Guide Book*, Mulford Biological Laboratories (of Sharp & Dohme), c. 1935, MA; Mufson, "Streptococcus Pneumoniae," p. 1543.

29 These bacteria belong to the streptococcus pneumoniae species. *Streptococcus pneumoniae* is a diploid, lancet-shaped, gram-positive bacterium. It possesses an outer polysaccharide capsule that varies distinctly from one form of bacterium to another. While a small number of this bacterium's serologic types cause the vast majority of the cases of pneumococcal disease, the major sources of infection have over the years shifted to new types. The capsular covering of this bacterium is, as it were, both a signature and a template. It contributes to the bacterium's virulence by helping to protect it from engulfment and digestion by phagocytic white blood cells. R. E. Weibel, P. P. Vella, A. A. McLean, A. F. Woodhour, W. L. Davidson, and M. R. Hilleman, "Studies in Human Subjects of Polyvalent Pneumococcal Vaccines," *Proceedings of the Society for Experimental Biology and Medicine* 156, no. 1 (1977): 144–50.

pneumococcal vaccine.[30] So had Squibb, but the company abandoned its two hexavalent pneumococcal polysaccharide vaccines (one for children, the other for adults) because it was unlikely that physicians would urge or public health organizations would pay for immunization against the disease.[31]

But Robert Austrian and his colleague Dr. Jerome Gold were persistent. They put together data from the Kings County Hospital in Brooklyn and found that over a third of the bacteremic pneumonia patients died within twenty-four hours of admission to the hospital. Even the best medicines could not take effect in that short time. They also showed that even with effective drug treatment, the death rates in the first five days of illness were high. Pathologic alterations had already determined the outcome. Their study, published in 1964, led to renewed interest in vaccines for this disease.[32] In January 1968, the National

---

30 Heidelberger and Avery – the latter, once Mulford's consultant; see Chapter 2, note 42 – discovered the complex capsular carbohydrates that determine the type of the pneumococcus. For background on the early efforts to develop whole-bacteria vaccines and on subsequent developments with capsular vaccines, see the following: G. D. Maynard, "Pneumonia Inoculation Experiment No. III," *Medical Journal of South Africa* 11 (1915): 36–8; F. S. Lister, "Prophylactic Inoculation of Man Against Pneumococcal Infections, and More Particularly Against Lobar Pneumonia," *Publications of the South African Institute for Medical Research* 10 (1917): 304–22; Mufson, "Streptococcus Pneumoniae," p. 1548; T. Francis and W. S. Tillet, "Cutaneous Reactions in Pneumonia: The Development of Antibodies Following the Intradermal Injection of Type-Specific Polysaccharide," *Journal of Experimental Medicine* 52, no. 4 (1930): 573; *New England Journal of Medicine* 298, no. 6 (1978): 343; Chase, *Magic Shots*, pp. 22–3.

31 *Nature* 221 (Jan. 11, 1969): 117. "History of Pneumococcal Research," pp. 9, 15–16, MA.

32 *Nature* 221 (Jan. 11, 1969): 117. The journal noted with a confidence characteristic of research professionals in these years, "A polyvalent vaccine for mass-vaccination of high-risk groups should be ready by 1970." See also Mufson, "Streptococcus Pneumoniae," p. 1539; *New England Journal of Medicine* 288, no. 22 (1973): 1173–80; 299, no. 14 (1978): 735–40, 770–1; and *JAMA* 230, no. 3 (1974): 409–13.

Institute of Allergy and Infectious Diseases began to support research aimed at developing an effective pneumococcal polysaccharide vaccine. The Institute's specific project was to determine which types of pneumococci were responsible for most of the infections and to prepare polysaccharides from these types for use in vaccines. Working under this contract, Eli Lilly and Austrian developed quadravalent and hexavalent vaccines.[33]

But the company had numerous production problems with the new product and then some of the Navajo children involved in one of the clinical trials developed severe local reactions to the vaccine. During these years, Lilly was reconsidering its entire vaccine operation. Like Merck, it was concerned about the economic aspects of vaccine work, and the problems with the pneumonia vaccine convinced the company to withdraw first from that project and then from vaccine research entirely.[34]

Merck had by that time already entered the scene. Working without federal financial support, Hilleman and Austrian had teamed up in 1970 to develop a new capsular vaccine. Many of the members of the Penn/Merck teams who had worked on influenza and respiratory diseases were also involved in this new round of research and clinical

33 R. Austrian, "Pneumococcal Infection," *Preventive Medicine* 3, no. 4 (1974): 443–5. See also Austrian's letter in *JAMA* 231, no. 4 (1975): 345–6; and *New England Journal of Medicine* 297, no. 17 (1977): 897–900.

34 In 1978, Lilly explained to Merck that it had decided to terminate all vaccine production except its rabies vaccine, for which it was the only supplier in the nation. The correspondent mentioned the considerations that guided the firm's decision: the market was not growing; there was considerable competition for the market in vaccines for childhood diseases; margins were tight; the R & D was expensive, as were the clinical and safety tests. In regard to the pneumonia vaccine in particular, the letter said: "Documenting the efficacy of a vaccine in the United States is difficult and expensive. This is especially true for diseases occurring at low incidence rates. The incidence of pneumococcal diseases was – and still is – difficult to assess, and accurate diagnostic techniques are expensive and difficult to perform." "History of Pneumococcal Research," pp. 10, 16–17; see also *Pneumovax* Backgrounder, MSD, p. 9; both in MA.

trials.[35] Hilleman had two separate groups working on this project, one at West Point, the other at Rahway.[36] The division of labor accurately indicated the complexity of the task. After Austrian provided the seed stock of most of the pneumococcal bacteria, the Rahway group grew the bacteria and isolated, purified, and tested each of the polysaccharides. Then West Point took over, formulating the purified polysaccharides into vaccines.[37]

West Point worked with the clinical teams that tested three experimental vaccines: one contained six pneumococcal types, another twelve, and the third fourteen.[38] The first clinical trials, which began in early 1973, involved nearly 13,000 adults and children. One of the

---

35 Weibel, Vella, McLean, Woodhour, Davidson, and Hilleman, "Studies in Human Subjects of Polyvalent Pneumococcal Vaccines," pp. 144–50.

36 Ibid. "History of Pneumococcal Research," p. 10, MA. The West Point contingent included Allen F. Woodhour, in addition to Vella and McLean. The Rahway group included T. Stoudt, D. J. Carlo, B. L. Wilker, K. Nollstadt, J. Wolski, and R. Walton.

37 The vaccine did not contain whole pneumococcal bacteria, but rather the highly purified capsular polysaccharides derived from the most prevalent or invasive pneumococcal types. To produce sufficient polysaccharide, the bacteria were grown in containers of ever-increasing size, beginning with small culture dishes and ending with 800-liter fermentation tanks. Once the growth cycle was completed, the bacteria were killed with phenol and separated from the fluid. M. R. Hilleman, "Notes," MA. Weibel, Vella, McLean, Woodhour, Davidson, and Hilleman, "Studies in Human Subjects of Polyvalent Pneumococcal Vaccines," pp. 144–50.

Purification was achieved by chemically removing the capsular material and subjecting it to a series of centrifugation and purification steps, monitored by antibody probe. The material was finally dried into a white powder. At each stage in the processing, the Merck team conducted tests to ensure the chemical purity of the carbohydrates. After they tested each of the separate, dried polysaccharides for identity, purity, toxicity, and amount, they combined them in solution and diluted them to the desired concentration.

38 Operating under the Investigative New Drug Regulations, Merck submitted to the government descriptions of each product, the test results, and the firm's clinical plans.

---

larger tests was performed among gold miners in the South African Transvaal. Laboring in arduous conditions of heat and humidity, these workers had long suffered high rates of pneumococcal pneumonia.[39] As the tests indicated, however, the new six- and twelve-valent vaccines were both effective, especially the latter.[40] The six-valent dose resulted in a 76 percent reduction in the incidence of pneumonia caused by the particular serotypes in the vaccine. For the twelve-valent dose, the reduction was 92 percent.[41]

The large number of serotypes and the inability to predict which would be dominant at a particular time complicated the clinical tests, as they did the problems of producing an effective vaccine. There is no cross-protection between the different types. So it was necessary in the clinical trials to perform a specific etiologic serotype diagnosis for each patient. By comparing attack rates in the vaccinated and control groups, the researchers could calculate protective efficacy.[42]

---

39 See the discussion in S. Lister and D. Ordman, "The Epidemiology of Pneumonia on the Witwatersrand Goldfields and the Prevention of Pneumonia and Other Allied Acute Respiratory Diseases in Native Labourers in South Africa by Means of Vaccine," *South African Institute for Medical Research* 7, no. 37 (1935): 1–81.

40 The vaccines were administered to 1,523 young men who had just arrived at the mines. A further 3,171 were included in the study as controls. Smit, Oberholzer, Hayden-Smith, Koornhoff, and Hilleman, "Protective Efficacy of Pneumococcal Polysaccharide Vaccines Against Pneumococcal Pneumonia," pp. 2613–16; see also *JAMA* 237, no. 24 (1977): 2605.

41 The reduction in each case was for the particular sereotypes included in the particular vaccine. These sereotypes covered a high percentage of the sources of infection. A. B. Kaiser and W. Schaffner, "Prospectus: The Prevention of Bacteremic Pneumococcal Pneumonia: A Conservative Appraisal of Vaccine Intervention," *JAMA* 230, no. 3 (1974): 404–8. See also I. D. Riley, M. Andrews, R. Howard, P. I. Tarr, M. Pfeiffer, P. Challands, and G. Jennison, "Immunisation with a Polyvalent Pneumococcal Vaccine," *Lancet* (June 25, 1977): 1338–41, for a report on clinical tests in New Guinea; and Robert Austrian's commentary in *JAMA* 297, no. 17 (1977): 938–9.

42 In clinical tests, it was possible to show protective efficacy for only a few of the serotypes. Preparation of a polyvalent vaccine was thus based on analogy. Anti-

The clinical teams also conducted tests of the twelve- and fourteen-valent vaccines closer to home, among open populations in the suburban Philadelphia area and among Merck employees. Again, the results were satisfying, with all but a few of the subjects displaying significant increases in antibodies and minimal clinical reactions.[43] By 1977, the company had substantial evidence of the vaccines' efficacy, and in November of that year, the U.S. government issued a license for the fourteen-valent *Pneumovax*.[44] At this stage, Merck could not assure long-term immunity, and very young children did not develop antibodies in an acceptable manner.[45] But following additional clinical tests and the development of a new twenty-three-serotype vaccine

---

body seroconversions were the markers of protection, and other serotypes producing similar antibody responses were presumed also to be effective. This presumption was validated in the large surveillance studies that followed the introduction of the vaccine for general use. M. R. Hilleman, "Notes," MA.

43 Weibel, Vella, McLean, Woodhour, Davidson, and Hilleman, "Studies in Human Subjects of Polyvalent Pneumococcal Vaccines," pp. 144–50.

44 In addition to conducting its own tests, Merck had sent large quantities of the vaccine to the NIAID for independent clinical studies. "History of Pneumococcal Research," p. 10; FDA press release, Nov. 1977; MSD press release, Nov. 23, 1977; *FDA Drug Bulletin* (1978): 4–5; all in MA.

45 The responsiveness of infants to the vaccine was important because pneumococci are a prime cause of otitis media. Hilleman worked with Dr. Helena Mäkelä in Finland in exploring this relationship. See *Lancet* (Sept. 13, 1980): 547–51; *Lancet* (Dec. 6, 1980): 1248–9; *Pediatric Infectious Disease Journal* 5, no. 1 (1986): 39–44, 45–50. See also *Pediatric Research* 18, no. 11 (1984): 1067–71. Researchers would be unable, however, to solve this problem until they learned how to couple polysaccharide to a protein carrier. See the discussion in this chapter. For children over two years of age, the vaccine was effective. *Pediatrics* 61, no. 2 (1978): 321–2. See also *New England Journal of Medicine* 299, no. 14 (1978): 778–9; 300, no. 3 (1979): 143; 300, no. 4 (1979): 203–4; *JAMA* 241, no. 18 (1979): 1935; 268, no. 23 (1992): 3323–7, 3328–32; and *Pediatrics* 62, no. 5 (1978): 721–7 – the latter for a report on a clinical trial with the Eli Lilly product. But see *Pediatric Infectious Disease Journal* 1, no. 1 (1982): 34–6; and *Pediatrics* 69, no. 2 (1982): 219–23; and 75, no. 6 (1985): 1153–8.

(*Pneumovax 23*, 1983), physicians could ensure long-term protection by giving booster shots to restore immunity.[46]

The pneumonia vaccine gave Merck a product with considerable potential for future development. After the distribution of about four million doses, *Pneumovax* was credited with excellent antibody responses among young as well as older adults.[47] The American population was aging, and with gerontology steadily becoming a more important specialty, the long-term prospects for Merck's new vaccine were

---

46 A. J. Carlson, W. L. Davidson, A. A. McLean, P. P. Vella, R. E. Weibel, A. F. Woodhour, and M. R. Hilleman, "Pneumococcal Vaccine: Dose, Revaccination, and Coadministration with Influenza Vaccine," *Proceedings of the Society for Experimental Biology and Medicine* 161 (1979): 558–63; see also *Proceedings of the Society for Experimental Biology and Medicine* 164 (1980): 435–8. M. R. Hilleman, A. A. McLean, P. P. Vella, R. E. Weibel, and A. F. Woodhour, "Polyvalent Pneumococcal Polysaccharide Vaccines," *Journal of Infection* 1, no. 2 (1979): 1–16; M. R. Hilleman, A. A. McLean, P. P. Vella, R. E. Weibel, and A. F. Woodhour, "Pneumococcal Vaccines," *Pathologie Biologie* 27, no. 9 (1979): 579–88; M. R. Hilleman, A. F. Woodhour, R. E. Weibel, P. P. Vella, A. A. McLean, and A. J. Carlson, Jr., "Vaccination Against Pneumococcal Infections," in H. P. Lambert and A. D. S. Caldwell, eds., *Pneumonia and Pneumococcal Infections*, Royal Society of Medicine International Congress and Symposium Series, no. 27 (London, 1980); M. R. Hilleman, A. F. Woodhour, R. E. Weibel, P. P. Vella, A. A. McLean, and A. J. Carlson, Jr., "Vaccine Prevention of Pneumococcal Diseases," *Medicina Clinica* 80, supp. 1 (1983): 30–40.

The number of types was crucial because the key element in pneumococcal vaccine is the manner in which it fills in for serotypes for which antibody is lacking. Most of us have antibody against most types, and disease only occurs when a specific serotype infection takes place in the absence of antibody. The vaccine provides protection by filling in the gaps.

47 M. R. Hilleman, A. J. Carlson, Jr., A. A. McLean, P. P. Vella, R. E. Weibel, and A. F. Woodhour, "Streptococcus Pneumoniae Polysaccharide Vaccine: Age and Dose Responses, Safety, Persistence of Antibody, Revaccination, and Simultaneous Administration of Pneumococcal and Influenza Vaccines," *Reviews of Infectious Diseases* 3, supp. (1981): S31–42.

good.[48] This was especially true because Robert Austrian had not given up his quest.[49] Through the 1980s, he continued his studies and publications calling for prevention, as did other healthcare professionals.[50]

48 On Merck's efforts to use the medical networks to develop interest in the new product see C. A. High to Philippe Blanc, May 4, 1979; High to R. Brice, et al., July 5, 1979; J. P. Salmela to R. Brice, et al., Jan. 30, 1980; R. D. Brice to J. W. Stuart, et al., Mar. 20, 1980; all in MA. It is not entirely clear why the response was not more decisive. One explanation is that the nation's medical care system was still oriented more to treatment of acute illness than to prevention – especially where older adults were concerned. Then too, Merck had originally established the efficacy of the new vaccine in populations outside of the United States. This raised questions for some healthcare professionals as to whether it would be equally effective among elderly Americans. See J. C. Butler, R. F. Breiman, J. F. Campbell, H. B. Lipman, C. V. Broome, and R. R. Facklam, "Pneumococcal Polysaccharide Vaccine Efficacy," *JAMA* 270, no. 15 (1993): 1826–31.

49 There were others calling for more vigorous efforts to promote immunization. R. H. Pantell and T. J. Stewart, "The Pneumococcal Vaccine: Immunization at a Crossroad," *JAMA* 241, no. 21 (1979): 2272–4, said that there was a "waning of interest" in disease prevention and an "information gap" about new vaccines like *Pneumovax*. An editorial (p. 2299) agreed that there was a problem. See also J. W. Shands, Jr., "What is the Role of Vaccines in Treating the Older Patient?" *Geriatrics* 34, no. 11 (1979): 62–5.

50 See, for instance, *JAMA* 243, no. 24 (1980): 2525; *Journal of the American Geriatrics Society* 29, no. 11 (1981): 481–9. G. O. Williams, "Vaccines in Older Patients: Combating the Risk of Mortality," *Geriatrics* 35, no. 11 (1980): 55–64; see also *Geriatrics* 37, no. 4 (1982): 65–78. Austrian complained in 1980 that the Centers for Disease Control and their Advisory Committee on Immunization Practices had "done little to encourage the administration of pneumococcal vaccine to adult populations who are at high risk of death from pneumococcal infection." *New England Journal of Medicine* 303, no. 10 (1980): 578–80. In the same issue see J. S. Willems, C. R. Sanders, M. A. Riddiough, and J. C. Bell, "Cost Effectiveness of Vaccination Against Pneumococcal Pneumonia," pp. 553–9. A similar cost-effectiveness study appears in *JAMA* 245, no. 5 (1981): 473–7; see also the editorial on pp. 498–9. See also *Pediatrics* 67, no. 4 (1981): 548–51; *JAMA* 245, no. 22 (1981): 2288; 246, no. 13 (1981): 1428–32; 249, no. 12 (1983): 1566–7; *Journal of the American Geriatrics Society* 29, no. 4 (1981): 181–5. *Geriatrics* 37, no. 10 (1982): 78–84.

Meanwhile, clinical trials indicated that the pneumonia and influenza vaccines could be administered at the same time.[51]

Nevertheless, the experts in the medical and research networks remained divided in this case, and that was a difficult situation for Merck – especially in a healthcare system in which third-party payment, and thus consensus on the part of medical professionals, was of decisive importance.[52] As late as 1984, immunization levels remained low. Austrian noted that "less than a quarter of patients recognized to be at high risk of death if infected have been immunized."[53] Two years later, the same story was repeated,[54] even though there was some evidence by this time that vaccination against this infection was "re-

51 F. DeStefano, R. A. Goodman, G. R. Noble, G. D. McClary, S. J. Smith, and C. V. Broome, "Simultaneous Administration of Influenza and Pneumococcal Vaccines," *JAMA* 247, no. 18 (1982): 2551–4. As of July 1981, pneumococcal vaccine immunization was covered under Medicare.

52 For an excellent discussion of the role in post-World War II American politics of experts and of conflicts within expert networks see Balogh, *Chain Reaction*. On the continued controversies in the 1990s see: *Lancet* (Apr. 14, 1990): 898–9; *Pediatric Infectious Disease Journal* 9, no. 4 (1990): 258–62; 10, no. 5 (1991): 386–90; *JAMA* 264, no. 9 (1990): 1117–22; 264, no. 22 (1990): 2910–15; 265, no. 17 (1991): 2193–4; 270, no. 15 (1993): 1826–31; 270, no. 22 (1993): 2735–6; *Journal of the American Geriatrics Society* 39, no. 1 (1991): 108–13; 42, no. 11 (1994): 1154–9; *Pediatrics* 88, no. 5 (1991): 1074–5; *New England Journal of Medicine* 325, no. 21 (1991): 1506–8; *Geriatrics* 48, no. 2 (1993): 43–50; 49, no. 11 (1994): 9; *Preventive Medicine* 23 (1994): 751–5.

53 R. Austrian, "A Reassessment of Pneumococcal Vaccine," *New England Journal of Medicine* 310, no. 10 (1984): 651–3. Austrian raised the possibility that the vaccine might become unavailable – for the second time! – if these conditions continued. The Centers for Disease Control recommended broader usage of the vaccine in 1984. *JAMA* 251, no. 23 (1984): 3071–5. See also the exchange in *JAMA* 311, no. 4 (1984): 260–1.

54 D. S. Fedson, "Improving the Use of Pneumococcal Vaccine Through a Strategy of Hospital-Based Immunization: A Review of Its Rationale and Implications," *Journal of the American Geriatrics Society* 33, no. 2 (1985): 142–50; see also 33, no. 3 (1985): 175–8.

gaining acceptance."[55] During this interlude, sales of *Pneumovax* and *Pneumovax 23* were growing, but the company recognized that it had fallen short of tapping the full potential for this new vaccine.[56] There was encouraging news in 1991, when Austrian and his coworkers – including researchers from Yale and the National Institute of Child Health and Human Development – announced the results of a new, hospital-based, case-control study among adults. Using both the fourteen- and twenty-three-valent vaccines, Austrian and his colleagues established the protective efficacy of the vaccines and concluded that they were the best means of preventing invasive pneumococcal infections.[57] The vaccine, they concluded, "should be used more widely." There was by this time considerable evidence that the medical, scientific, and public health networks were moving toward consensus – at least in the United States – a development that would provide additional confirmation of Merck's decision in the 1970s to take a long-

---

55 S. L. Berk and S. Alvarez, "Vaccinating the Elderly: Recommendations and Rationale," *Geriatrics* 41, no. 1 (1986): 79–91. See also *Geriatrics* 41, no. 5 (1986): 101–2; 41, no. 11 (1986): 13–16; 42, no. 10 (1987): 81–90; 44, no. 8 (1989): 66; and *Journal of the American Geriatrics Society* 35, no. 8 (1987): 747–54; 36, no. 10 (1988): 897–901. *JAMA* 261, no. 9 (1989): 1265–7.

56 Merck's only competitor in the United States was Lederle Laboratories, which had developed Pnu-Immune 23. Pasteur-Mérieux-Connaught marketed Pneumo 23 in Europe. But SmithKline Beecham had withdrawn its seventeen-valent vaccine from the market in 1988. D. S. Fedson and D. M. Musher, "Pneumococcal Vaccine," in Plotkin and Mortimer, *Vaccines*, p. 532. Between 1978 and 1991, twenty-three million doses were sold in the United States and around 20 percent of the nation's elderly persons were vaccinated (ibid., p. 547).

57 E. D. Shapiro, A. T. Berg, R. Austrian, D. Schroeder, V. Parcells, A. Margolis, R. K. Adair, and J. D. Clemens, "The Protective Efficacy of Polyvalent Pneumococcal Polysaccharide Vaccine," *New England Journal of Medicine* 325, no. 21 (1991): 1453–60. But for a contrary conclusion see *New England Journal of Medicine* 315, no. 21 (1986): 1318–27. See the response in *Journal of the American Geriatrics Society* 35, no. 4 (1987): 373–4; and the exchange in *New England Journal of Medicine* 316, no. 20 (1987): 1272–3.

range perspective on the potential of this field and to develop new bacterial vaccines.[58]

3

That same perspective would be needed with the third program Virus and Cell Biology launched in this second phase of vaccine innovation. The organization had by now acquired substantial capabilities in the area of bacterial vaccines, and it set out to apply that expertise against one of the major causes of death among children, bacterial meningitis.[59] By administering antibiotics, physicians have been able to save the lives of most children with this disease. But resistance had developed to a large number of the antibiotics, including ampicillin, the primary therapy for the disease.[60] Even with appropriate treatment, about 5 percent of those who developed *H. influenzae* Type b meningitis (HIB) died and approximately 15 to 30 percent were left with complications. HIB was a leading cause of acquired mental retardation in the United States, and the incidence and mortality from the disease were similar to those for polio *before* immunization was possible.[61]

First identified and reported in 1892 (Richard Pfeiffer in Germany), HIB was mistakenly hailed as the primary cause of influenza and was later thought to be responsible for the great flu pandemic of 1918–19. As researchers later learned, six strains of the bacteria have outer coatings (that is, capsules) that are of clinical

---

58 The best guide is Fedson and Musher, "Pneumococcal Vaccine," pp. 517–64.

59 There were, however, some cases in adults. See *New England Journal of Medicine* 282, no. 4 (1970): 190–4, 221–2; and 285, no. 12 (1971): 666–7.

60 A. L. Smith, "Antibiotics and Invasive *Haemophilus Influenzae*," *New England Journal of Medicine* 294, no. 24 (1976): 1329–31. *Pediatrics* 71, no. 2 (1983): 187–91. *Pediatric Infectious Disease Journal* 6, no. 8 (1987): 719–21.

61 J. Ward, J. M. Lieberman, and S. L. Cochi, "Haemophilus Influenzae Vaccines," in Plotkin and Mortimer, eds., *Vaccines*, pp. 337–86. See also *Pediatrics* 71, no. 6 (1983): 927–31.

significance in terms of virulence. The different capsules are used in serotyping strains a through f, two of which (a and b) cause disease.[62] Indigenous to humans, HIB is normally found in the pharynx and the pulmonary system and an estimated 80 percent of the population are carriers. Most are colonized with unencapsulated strains, but 3 to 5 percent are carrying strains with capsules – most often serotype b.[63]

Children are at the greatest risk from systemic infections. In many countries HIB meningitis exceeds the number of cases of disease caused by all other bacteria put together. It is a common cause of bacterial pneumonia. Nontypeable strains have been increasingly recognized over the last three decades as the agents most frequently responsible for otitis media in children.[64] In 1972, Dr. Sarah W. Sell and associates at Vanderbilt University Medical School published a devastating testimony to the permanent damage that could result from HIB meningitis. They had studied eighty-six children who had been treated with antibiotics during an acute outbreak in Nashville, Tennessee: eleven had died; twenty-six were left with severe handicaps; twelve had possible residual damage; and only thirty-seven were cured without residual problems. The handicaps included serious mental retardation, partial paralysis, seizures, partial blindness, and hearing, speech, and

62 J. B. Robbins and R. Schneerson, *"Haemophilus Influenzae* Type B: The Search for a Vaccine," *Pediatric Infectious Disease Journal* 6, no. 8 (1987): 791–4.

63 E. R. Moxon, "Haemophilus Influenzae," in Mandell, Douglas, and Bennett, eds., *Infectious Diseases*, p. 1723. The microorganism is a small, nonmotile, nonspore-forming, gram-negative bacterium that varies in form. Although it is a facultative anaerobe, it is aerobically cultured on a medium containing hemoglobin, which accounts for its generic name *Haemophilus* – that is, blood-loving. See also *Pediatric Research* 9 (1975): 513–16.

64 Moxon, "Haemophilus Influenzae," p. 1723. *Haemophilus Influenzae Type B, Medical Background*, section 1, pp. 7–11, MA. This disease is the chief cause among children of pyogenic meningitis, bacterial epiglottitis, bronchopulmonary infections, and bacteremic infections. The complications include cellulitis and pericarditis, sinusitis, and septic arthritis.

behavioral disorders. The high morbidity rates prompted a search for preventive medicine.[65]

At Merck, the company's research teams initially followed the research path used for *Pneumovax* and developed a vaccine from a purified capsular polysaccharide. The clinical studies indicated, however, that it had only about 70 percent efficacy and that it elicited little or no antibody response in children under two.[66] Nevertheless, three other companies continued down this path and developed polysaccharide capsular vaccines (identified as PRP, for polysaccharide polyribosylribitol phosphate) that the government licensed in 1985. The American Academy of Pediatrics and the U.S. Public Health Service recommended a single dose for all children at twenty-four months of age.[67]

---

65 S. H. W. Sell, R. E. Merrill, E. O. Doyne, and E. P. Zimsky, Jr., "Long-Term Sequelae of *Haemophilus Influenzae* Meningitis," *Pediatrics* 49, no. 2 (1972): 206–11. Chase, *Magic Shots*, pp. 36, 383–4. See also *Pediatric Infectious Disease Journal* 7, no. 4 (1988): 250–4. But see the commentary in *New England Journal of Medicine* 301, no. 3 (1979): 155–6, and the radically different results in 323, no. 24 (1990): 1657–63.

66 See J. C. Parke, Jr., R. Schneerson, J. B. Robbins, and J. Schlesselman, "Interim Report of a Controlled Field Trial of Immunization with Capsular Polysaccharides of *H. Influenzae* Type B and Group C *Neisseria Meningitidis* in Mecklenburg County, North Carolina," *Journal of Infectious Diseases* 136, supp. (1977): S51–6. See also *Pediatric Research* 7 (1973): 103–10; and *Pediatrics* 52, no. 5 (1973): 633–5, 637–44; 60, no. 5 (1977): 730–7, which reports on a large field study in Finland; 74, no. 5 (1984): 857–65; 77, no. 3 (1986): 289–95; *JAMA* 230, no. 10 (1974): 1458; *Preventive Medicine* 3 (1974): 446–8; *New England Journal of Medicine* 292, no. 21 (1975): 1093–6; 310, no. 24 (1984): 1561–6, 1595–6; 312, no. 1 (1985): 53–4; *Pediatric Infectious Disease Journal* 1, no. 2 (1982): 132–8.

67 The three companies were Praxis, Connaught Laboratories, and Lederle Laboratories. Ward, Lieberman, and Cochi, "Haemophilus Influenzae Vaccines," pp. 353, 356. *Lancet* (Oct. 3, 1981): 705–9. See also *JAMA* 253, no. 4 (1985): 521–9, for a cost-effectiveness study (positive) on the polysaccharide vaccine (PRP), and pp. 554–6, for an editorial on these developments; also 253, no. 9 (1985): 1232–3; 253, no. 18 (1985): 2630, 2636–7; 253, no. 21 (1985):

Although the companies sold nearly ten million doses of PRP-HIB and adverse reactions were rare, the vaccine would not protect the population at greatest risk — children under two.[68] Merck had continued to work on this central problem, and the solution came to Virus and Cell Biology by way of southern Portugal (the Algarve), where Hilleman attended a conference. By that time, the immunologists had separated blood lymphocytes into two groups: B cells that produced antibodies and T cells that gave help to B cells in making antibody. In children over two years old, B cells did not need T-cell help in eliciting antibodies, but this was not the case with most children under two. As an immunologist at the meeting reported, however, he was able to elicit a T helper response in very young animals by coupling polysaccharide to a carrier protein. "This was an electrifying revelation — a revolutionary event in science," Hilleman later observed. "It opened a door," enabling Merck to solve "the problem of infant immunization."[69]

Merck immediately started a coupling program and carried this work forward under the leadership of Dr. Edward Scolnick, the

---

3063; and 257, no. 23 (1987): 3182–3. *Pediatric Infectious Disease Journal* 4, no. 4 (1985): 355–7; 6, no. 1 (1987): 6–7, 20–3. *Pediatrics* 76, no. 2 (1985): 322–4.

The decision by the American Academy of Pediatrics, Committee on Infectious Diseases, and the Immunization Practices Advisory Committee to recommend immunization for all children at twenty-four months of age prompted some concern. See *Pediatrics* 77, no. 2 (1986): 258–60; 79, no. 3 (1987): 321–5; 80, no. 2 (1987): 270–4; 81, no. 6 (1988): 886–97; 84, no. 2 (1989): 255–61. *New England Journal of Medicine* 315, no. 25 (1986): 1584–90. See also *Pediatric Infectious Disease Journal* 6, no. 7 (1987): 660–5; 7, no. 3 (1988): 147–8, 149–56; 7, no. 8 (1988): 574–7. *Military Medicine* 154, no. 1 (1989): 25–9. *JAMA* 261, no. 8 (1989): 1152–3; 261, no. 13 (1989): 1924–9.

68 See, for instance, *Pediatrics* 79, no. 2 (1987): 173–80; 80, no. 3 (1987): 319–29. *Pediatric Infectious Disease Journal* 6, no. 3 (1987): 305; and 6, no. 8 (1987): 795–8.

69 M. R. Hilleman, "Notes," MA.

---

new head of Virus and Cell Biology.[70] Hilleman, who retired in 1984, remained actively involved as a consultant. But Scolnick now had to make the crucial decisions about the HIB program, which had by this time found a protein to use for coupling. They were employing one from the outer coat of meningococcus B, a protein that the Behringwerke firm in Marburg, Germany, had isolated in abundance and patented with other uses in mind. Merck licensed this protein for its new project.[71] Even with the protein in hand, the coupling program was complex and time-consuming. Virus and Cell Biology turned to Merck's organic chemists (under Dr. Burton G. Christensen), who after considerable effort developed covalent coupling reactions that were predictable, controllable, and precisely directed. They linked a protein carrier with a polysaccharide hapten, a partial antigen, of

---

70 Dr. Scolnick received his M.D. from the Harvard Medical School in 1965. Following internship and residency at Massachusetts General Hospital, he joined the National Heart Institute, where he worked on protein synthesis. In 1970, he joined the National Cancer Institute as Senior Staff Fellow and became head of the Institute's Genetics Section the next year. His research at the Institute demonstrated the cellular origin of sarcoma virus oncogenes in mammals and defined specific genes that are implicated in human malignant disease. He was the author or coauthor of 176 scientific publications and won the Arthur S. Flemming Award (1976), the Public Health Service Superior Service Award (1978), and the Eli Lilly Award in Microbiology (1980). In 1982, Scolnick became executive director of basic research in Virus and Cell Biology; the following year, he became vice president and director of that department. He also served as editor-in-chief of *The Journal of Virology* from 1982 to 1985.

71 M. R. Hilleman, "Notes," MA. Connaught was using diphtheria toxoid for coupling. *Lancet* (May 25, 1985): 1184–6; and *Lancet* (May 10, 1986): 1074–5. Tetanus toxoid was also being used. S. L. Cochi and C. V. Broome, "Vaccine Prevention of *Haemophilus Influenzae* Type B Disease: Past, Present and Future," *Pediatric Infectious Disease Journal* 5, no. 1 (1986): 12–19. Merck was concerned, however, that repeated use of a single protein might induce tolerance and nonresponsiveness. With this in mind, Virus and Cell Biology steered away from proteins used to immunize against diphtheria or tetanus. See also *New England Journal of Medicine* 315, no. 8 (1986): 499–503; and *Pediatric Infectious Disease Journal* 6, no. 8 (1987): 804–7.

HIB.[72] After treating the conjugate – that is, the linked protein and polysaccharide – they lyophilized it for storage.[73]

Merck's initial clinical studies were successful. The first, involving ten healthy adults, resulted in no adverse reactions; that was also the case in a subsequent trial with thirty-one children in suburban Philadelphia. Because certain ethnic groups – including Native Americans – are particularly susceptible to HIB, the company conducted a large clinical study among Navajo infants. This study confirmed both the efficacy and safety of the vaccine, which stimulated high levels of antibody production.[74]

In December 1989, the government licensed *PedvaxHIB*, the third HIB conjugate vaccine to come on the American market.[75] At

---

72 The MSDRL research team – with support from Dr. Edward M. Scolnick and Dr. S. Marburg – grew its strain of *H. influenzae* Type b (the Ross strain, which had been obtained from the State University of New York) in supplemented heart infusion broth.

73 At each stage, the lots were subjected to the rabbit pyrogen test, using specifications set for meningococcal polysaccharides. Antibody titers for the vaccine were determined by radioimmunoassay from mouse potency and human clinical trials.

74 J. Y. Tai, P. P. Vella, A. A. McLean, A. F. Woodhour, W. J. McAleer, A. Sha, C. Dennis-Sykes, and M. R. Hilleman, *"Haemophilus Influenzae* Type B Polysaccharide-Protein Conjugate Vaccine," *Proceedings of the Society for Experimental Biology and Medicine* 184 (1987): 154–61. A. A. Lenoir, P. D. Granoff, and D. M. Granoff, "Immunogenicity of *Haemophilus Influenzae* Type B Polysaccharide-*Neisseria Meningitidis* Outer Membrane Protein Conjugate Vaccine in 2- to 6-Month-Old Infants," *Pediatrics* 80, no. 2 (1987): 283–7. Merck sponsored the April 1990 supplement to *Pediatrics* 85, no. 4, which was devoted to HIB vaccines. Several of the contributors presented results of clinical trials using Merck's new conjugate vaccine (identified as PRP-OMV, for Outer Membrane Protein). See also *Pediatric Research* 24, no. 2 (1988): 180–5, and the commentary in *Pediatric Infectious Disease Journal* 6, no. 8 (1987): 799–803. See also *JAMA* 261, no. 14 (1989): 2015, 2019.

75 The first, in December 1987, was Connaught's PRP-D vaccine (polysaccharide linked to a diphtheria toxoid carrier) for the age group eighteen to fifty-nine months, and later fifteen to fifty-nine months. The second, in December 1988,

---

first, the approval was for use in children over the age of eighteen months, but the following year, this was changed to two months and older.[76] *PedvaxHIB* was "unique among the HIB conjugate vaccines in its ability to induce a strong antibody response in young infants with the first dose."[77] Wherever they have been used extensively, the

---

was Praxis/Lederle's HbOC vaccine (oligosaccharides linked to a nontoxic diphtheria toxin) for the age group eighteen to fifty-nine months, and later fifteen to fifty-nine months. Ward, Lieberman, and Cochi, "Haemophilus Influenzae Vaccines," pp. 353, 356–64. *Pediatrics* 80, no. 3 (1987): 351–4; 81, no. 6 (1988): 908–11; 82, no. 4 (1988): 571–5; 83, no. 1 (1989): 145–6; 84, no. 2 (1989): 386–7; 84, no. 6 (1989): 995–9; 85, no. 3 (1990): 288–93, 331–7. *JAMA* 259, no. 5 (1988): 643–4; 259, no. 6 (1988): 798, 803–4; 261, no. 8 (1989): 1118. *Pediatric Infectious Disease Journal* 7, no. 3 (1988): 156–9; 8, no. 5 (1989): 297–302; 8, no. 8 (1989): 508–11; 8, no. 12 (1989): 883–4. *Military Medicine* 155, no. 10 (1990): 483–6. *Pediatric Research* 27, no. 4 (1990): 358-64.

76 Initially, Merck's only competition in the two months and older group of children was the Praxis/Lederle product; later, Connaught and SmithKline Beecham had vaccines approved for this age group. Ward, Lieberman, and Cochi, "Haemophilus Influenzae Vaccines," pp. 353, 362–6. *JAMA* 263, no. 18 (1990): 2429; 264, no. 2 (1990): 164; 264, no. 11 (1990): 1375; 264, no. 18 (1990): 2372. E. D. Shapiro, "New Vaccines Against *Haemophilus Influenzae* Type B," *Pediatric Clinics of North America* 37, no. 3 (1990): 567–83. *Pediatrics* 86, no. 1 (1990): 102–7; 86, no. 5 (1990): 794–6. *Pediatric Infectious Disease Journal* 9, no. 9 (1990): 632–5. Tai, Vella, McLean, Woodhour, McAleer, Sha, Dennis-Sykes, and Hilleman, "*Haemophilus Influenzae* Type B Polysaccharide-Protein Conjugate Vaccine," pp. 154–61. *Haemophilus Influenzae Type B, Medical Background*, section 4, pp. 3–6, MA. Moxon, "Haemophilus Influenzae," pp. 1727–8. See also *Pediatric Infectious Disease Journal* 9, no. 8 (1990): 555–61, and *New England Journal of Medicine* 323, no. 20 (1990): 1381-7, 1393–1401, and 1415–16, on Connaught's product. See *Pediatrics* 86, no. 4 (1990): 34, on the Praxis/Lederle vaccine.

77 Ward, Lieberman, and Cochi, "Haemophilus Influenzae Vaccines," p. 364. The antibody response after two doses of *PedvaxHIB* was higher than it was for the other vaccines. Merck encountered problems between August 1990 and May 1992 with sixteen lots of vaccine that were less immunogenic than its standard preparation and revaccination was recommended. Since 1992, the company has not experienced this problem. See also *World Health Organization Drug Information* 4, no. 4 (1990): 160.

conjugate vaccines – including Merck's – have practically eliminated HIB disease. By 1991, more than seventeen million doses were being sold or distributed each year in the United States alone, and there was a solid consensus in the medical and scientific networks about the need for even more extensive vaccination in the United States and abroad.[78]

While *PedvaxHIB* and *Pneumovax* were not yet important commercial products for Merck, they were significant indicators that Virus and Cell Biology was not locked on one course. The organization was still able to broaden its capabilities. This is one of the ways organizations that remain innovative over the long term are able to deal with long-cycle transitions. In this case, forceful science management nudged the research organization toward a new innovative pathway. The polysaccharide-capsule cycle would be neither as long nor as fruitful as the virology cycle had been, but it gave a new burst of energy to Merck's vaccine operations in the 1970s and 1980s.

4

As Merck was completing its first round of clinical tests with *PedvaxHIB*, the long-awaited multinetwork, nonprofit/private-sector/ public-sector, three-pronged study of innovation in vaccines was at last completed. The timing was exquisite. One wing of the project, which had been formally launched in 1980, employed a behavioral, "combined cost-effectiveness/decision" model that used quantitative data to

---

78 On the impact of the vaccines see Ward, Lieberman, and Cochi, "*Haemophilus Influenzae* Vaccines," pp. 368–70; *JAMA* 269, no. 2 (1993): 221–6, 227–31, 246–8, 264–6. The study by W. G. Adams, K. A. Deaver, S. L. Cochi, B. D. Plikaytis, E. R. Zell, C. V. Broome, and J. D. Wenger, "Decline of Childhood *Haemophilus Influenzae* Type B (Hib) Disease in the Hib Vaccine Era," *JAMA* 269, no. 2 (1993): 221–6, concluded that the vaccines had prevented "an estimated 10,000 to 16,000 cases of Hib disease in 1991."

On the need to encourage greater use of the vaccine see *Pediatrics* 80, no. 2 (1987): 288–9; 81, no. 1 (1988): 166–8. See *Pediatric Infectious Disease Journal* 9, no. 4 (1990): 246–51, for a cost-benefit study.

develop national priorities.[79] Vaccines were ranked according to: (1) the expected health benefits to be achieved by reducing morbidity and mortality; and (2) the anticipated net savings of healthcare resources. Using quantitative data, this model was applied to fourteen diseases important in the United States. It yielded the top five priorities: hepatitis B; respiratory syncytial virus (RSV); *H. influenzae* Type b; influenza; and *Herpesvirus varicellae* (for high-risk individuals). After five years of research, this formidable, government-sponsored study concluded that the HIB vaccine was a high-priority need – just as the new conjugate vaccines against HIB were about to become widely available to American children.[80]

A second and complementary wing of the Institute of Medicine's study was more productive.[81] The Institute's Committee on Public-Private Sector Relations in Vaccine Innovation eschewed formal modeling and used an historical-institutional approach to what it perceived as a major national problem: "more than half of the vaccine

---

79 The analytical approach, the researchers stated bluntly, was "reductionist: each logical component of expected benefits and of expected costs is assessed separately, then the components are aggregated in a stepwise fashion for each disease-vaccine contender." Institute of Medicine, Committee on Issues and Priorities for Vaccine Development, *New Vaccine Development: Establishing Priorities*, 1:28–38 provides an "Overview of the Analytic Approach."

80 By this time, Merck also already had its first hepatitis B vaccine on the market. In addition to the fine contrast between politically oriented and market-oriented performance, the study yielded an interesting paradox: originally launched in an effort to give the federal government a greater role in directing vaccine innovation (in the spirit of industrial policy), the project published its conclusions in the middle of the 1980s, when the government had turned away from industrial policy and toward a greater reliance on market-oriented, private-sector activity.

81 The third part of this project used the priority model for analyzing vaccine development for the underdeveloped nations. Institute of Medicine, Committee on Issues and Priorities for New Vaccine Development, *New Vaccine Development: Establishing Priorities*, vol. 2, *Diseases of Importance in Developing Countries*. We discuss this study and its impact in Chapter 8.

producers in the United States ceased production," the Committee noted, in the years 1968 through 1977. The decline had continued into the 1980s. With that change came a falloff in the level of private-sector support for vaccine innovation. While correctly observing that it was more difficult in vaccines than in pharmaceuticals to achieve patent protection, the Committee reached no conclusion about the obvious impact on profits of bulk government purchases with low margins.[82] Instead of dealing directly with that politically dangerous question, the Committee focused most of its attention on the liability problem. It urged "political decision makers to develop a compensation system for vaccine-related injury." The Committee wanted "to reduce the serious deterrents to vaccine manufacturing and innovation that arise from the unpredictable nature of the current liability situation."[83] These efforts would bear fruit in 1986, when Congress passed and President Reagan signed the National Childhood Vaccine Injury Act. This law fell short of providing the protection biological manufacturers wanted, but it represented a significant improvement in the existing legal situation for producers of pediatric vaccines.[84]

The new legal setting was important to Merck, but it was less important to Dr. Vagelos than the performance of the company's Virus and Cell Biology research. Now Chief Executive Officer of the world's leading pharmaceutical firm, Vagelos had already rejected the style of static cost-benefit analysis embodied in the Institute's priori-

---

82 Institute of Medicine, Division of Health Promotion and Disease Prevention, *Vaccine Supply and Innovation*, pp. 4–7, 45–64.

83 Ibid., pp. 12–13.

84 E. W. Kitch and E. A. Mortimer, Jr., "American Law, Preventive Vaccine Programs, and the National Vaccine Injury Compensation Program," in Plotkin and Mortimer, eds., *Vaccines*, especially pp. 939–41. The array of medical and biological professionals calling for federal action was impressive, both at the national and at the local/state levels. The Institute of Medicine study was just one part of that broad campaign, but it was an authoritative part with a broad geographical as well as professional representation.

ties.[85] Although concerned about the bottom line in 1979, he had opted instead for standards heavily weighted toward the medical benefits ensuing from successful innovation in all phases of the company's business.[86] By those standards the results of the bacterial-vaccine phase of Virus and Cell Biology R & D were unambiguous and positive. *Pneumovax* and *PedvaxHIB* were exactly the kinds of products Vagelos thought Merck should be producing and marketing. He was concerned about the manner in which the vaccine operation handled marketing and follow-up clinical studies, and he could see that Merck was not ideally positioned for the new age of combination vaccines that was emerging. But he was determined to improve the company's global position in this area of preventive medicine and to build on the substantial capabilities Virus and Cell Biology now had in bacterial as well as viral vaccines. He was especially pleased by the progress Merck had made in developing a vaccine against one of the world's most widespread diseases, hepatitis B.

85 Vagelos became CEO of Merck & Co., Inc., in July 1985, when John J. Horan retired. Vagelos would become chairman of Merck's board in April 1986 and would continue to serve in both positions until June 1994, when Raymond V. Gilmartin would become president and CEO of the firm. Vagelos would retire as chairman of the board on November 1, 1994.

86 Because the market was adequately supplied by Merck's competitors, Vagelos did not block the decisions to stop production of *Fluax* and *Meningovax*.

CHAPTER 8

NEW NETWORKS, NEW LEADERSHIP
THE HEPATITIS VACCINES

W HILE Virus and Cell Biology was developing new capabilities in bacterial vaccines, the department and Maurice Hilleman, its lead scientist for more than twenty-five years, had continued to explore the opportunities for new vaccines against viral infections.[1] One of the most important of these was hepatitis B (HBV), a virus with perhaps as many as 300 million long-term carriers around the world.[2] The first phase of this project lasted for thirteen years (1968–81) and the second, overlapping phase for eleven years (1975-86). This second phase of research and development carried Merck into contact with new scientific networks and forced the firm to develop entirely new capabilities. This transition took place against the backdrop of dramatic changes in leadership: in Virus and Cell Biology; at the Merck Sharp & Dohme Research Laboratories; and at the top of the corporation.

Substantial transitions in executive and scientific leadership can easily disrupt an organization's innovative process. This is espe-

---

1 Among the projects underway during these years were explorations of possible vaccines for respiratory syncytial virus (RSV), herpes simplex (types 1 and 2), and cytomegalovirus.

2 The estimates vary. See S. Krugman and C. E. Stevens, "Hepatitis B Vaccine," in Plotkin and Mortimer, eds., *Vaccines*, p. 425. Also W. S. Robinson, "Hepatitis B Virus and Hepatitis Delta Virus," in Mandell, Douglas, and Bennett, eds., *Infectious Diseases*, p. 1215.

cially true when a dominant leader like Hilleman has played a central role in creating and developing the company's scientific and technical capabilities. Customary patterns of teamwork are disturbed. The informal hierarchy that makes innovative organizations run successfully is disrupted, as are the important relationships to the external networks from which the business draws ideas, resources, and support. As we saw in the previous chapters, those relationships had important personal dimensions that were not easy to duplicate. In the worst-case scenario, a transformation in leadership can bring an end to a long cycle of successful innovation of the sort that had characterized the vaccine operations at Merck since the early 1960s.

So once again – in the 1980s, as in the previous decade – Merck's vaccine enterprise was at risk. The changes were clustered in the middle of the decade. Hilleman retired at the age of sixty-five. He was replaced by an outstanding scientist whose background was in basic, not applied, virology and who had before joining Merck shown no unusual interest in vaccines.[3] After only two years in this position, Dr. Edward M. Scolnick became president of MSDRL and acquired a broad range of new responsibilities. Scolnick replaced Dr. P. Roy Vagelos, who became CEO of Merck. There was cause for concern in that transition as well. Like Scolnick, Vagelos was a brilliant scientist and he had vigorously supported the vaccine operations in the past. But he was a self-acknowledged newcomer to business, had never taken a college course on any aspect of business, and had virtually no experience as a line officer running a large-scale organization. Given the number of unknowns in these organizational equations, the vaccine business at Merck was at best likely to experience major changes.

---

3 Dr. Edward Scolnick began at Merck in 1982 as executive director of basic research in the department of Virus and Cell Biology Research. In June 1983, Merck promoted him to director of the department and vice president, and he overlapped for a time with Hilleman, who did not retire until 1984. Hilleman continued to consult with the department and to take an active role in its programs after his retirement.

At worst, the enterprise might follow the pattern set at Eli Lilly and other major pharmaceutical firms that had abandoned vaccine research entirely.[4]

1

If Vagelos was able to hold the business on a course similar to the one he had set as president of MSDRL, the best argument for Virus and Cell Biology would be the kind of research and development it had been doing since the late 1960s on a vaccine against hepatitis. Viral hepatitis is caused by several agents and was doubtless the cause of what became known as yellow jaundice, an infection of the liver.[5] Military populations were especially prone to epidemics of jaundice, a disease whose viral etiology was not understood until the twentieth century.[6]

During World War II, epidemiological and human volunteer studies enabled researchers to separate hepatitis A – then known as "infectious hepatitis" – and hepatitis B – then known as "serum hepati-

<hr>

4 See the general discussion in P. L. Robertson and R. N. Langlois, "Institutions, Inertia and Changing Industrial Leadership," *Industrial and Corporate Change* 3, no. 2 (1994): 359–78.

5 These agents include hepatitis A virus (HAV), hepatitis B virus (HBV), the endemic, serum-transmitted, non-A and non-B hepatitis viruses (hepatitis C and possibly other, similar forms), the HBV-associated delta agent (HDV), and epidemic food- and water-borne non-A, non-B hepatitis virus. E. Robinson, "Hepatitis B Virus and Hepatitis Delta Virus," pp. 1204–14. F. B. Hollinger and A. P. Glombicki, "Hepatitis A Virus," in Mandell, Douglas, and Bennett, eds., *Infectious Diseases*, pp. 1383–7. S. M. Feinstone, "Non-A, Non-B Hepatitis," in Mandell, Douglas, and Bennett, eds., *Infectious Diseases*, pp. 1407–11. M. R. Hilleman, "Notes," MA.

6 *New England Journal of Medicine* 316, no. 16 (1987): 965–70. The incidence of hepatitis B was also high in prison populations. H. F. Hull, L. H. Lyons, J. M. Mann, S. C. Hadler, R. Steece, and M. R. Skeels, "Incidence of Hepatitis B in the Penitentiary of New Mexico," *American Journal of Public Health* 75, no. 10 (1985): 1134–5, 1182–5, 1213–14.

<hr>

183

tis."[7] At military bases in both World War II and the Korean War, there were repeated outbreaks of "serum hepatitis," with substantial morbidity and mortality. As recently as 1980, in fact, hepatitis B was the fifth most commonly reported infectious disease in the United States.[8] In the 1970s and early 1980s, the incidence of reported acute hepatitis B infections rose steadily,[9] and the Institute of Medicine ranked it at the top of the 1985 priority list for vaccine development.[10] Certain population groups are at particularly high risk, including healthcare workers, promiscuous persons in the homosexual community, and anyone exposed to human body fluids — including hemophiliacs and intravenous drug users who share needles.[11]

----

7 In 1883, hepatitis B had been reported as the cause of a jaundice epidemic among German shipyard workers who had received smallpox vaccinations containing human lymph. Thereafter, there were regular accounts of hepatitis B resulting from the use of contaminated needles, from the administration of human plasma, and from vaccines containing human serum (such as the yellow fever vaccine). Hence the name "serum hepatitis." During World War II, the Rockefeller Institute encountered this problem with a yellow fever vaccine its researchers had developed. Krugman and Stevens, "Hepatitis B Vaccine," p. 419.

8 W. D. Hillis, "Viral Hepatitis: An Unconquered Foe," *Military Medicine* 133, no. 5 (1968): 343–54. Chase, *Magic Shots*, pp. 275, 331–7. W. S. Robinson, "Hepatitis B Virus and Hepatitis Delta Virus," pp. 1204–31.

9 S. Krugman, "The Newly Licensed Hepatitis B Vaccine," *JAMA* 247, no. 14 (1982): 2012–15.

10 Institute of Medicine, Committee on Issues and Priorities, *New Vaccine Development: Establishing Priorities*, 1:129. Hepatitis B ranked first under three conditions: (1) if resource cost was not a consideration; (2) if resource cost was of secondary concern but $3.2 million dollars was considered excessive to save an "infant mortality equivalent"; and (3) if resource cost was of sufficient concern that even $125,000 was too much to save an "infant mortality equivalent." The infant mortality equivalent (IME) was explained as follows: "The IME value of a morbidity category/age group combination was calculated by multiplying the trade-off value assigned to a death in that age group compared to the death of an infant under one year of age" (p. 40).

11 *Journal of the American Geriatrics Society* 40, no. 3 (1992): 218–20. *Lancet* (July 17, 1982): 146–8; and *Lancet* (Oct. 2, 1982): 776. Chase, *Magic Shots*, pp. 331–

The frequency of the disease varies substantially around the world, with the lowest levels in Western Europe, the United States, and Australia, and the highest levels in Asia, Africa, and certain parts of the Middle East. In less developed countries, the disease is endemic, and even in the United States as many as 300,000 people – mainly young adults – become infected annually.[12] About 50,000 of these develop jaundice, 10,000 require hospitalization, and around 250 die. While approximately 90 percent of the patients with acute hepatitis make a full recovery, the remainder suffer from what may become serious complications.[13] Among the chronically infected population and carriers, the disease often progresses into cirrhosis or liver cancer. In the less developed countries about one-quarter of those chronically infected die from cirrhosis or hepatocellular carcinoma.[14]

---

2. The virus can be transmitted either *horizontally* (that is, from one individual in the population to another) or *vertically* (that is, from mother to fetus or neonate infant). Some individuals – who usually are asymptomatic – become chronically infected with HBV and are carriers. Newborns and young children infected with the virus are at far higher risk of becoming carriers than older persons. Of the babies born to carrier mothers, up to 90 percent may become carriers themselves. See also *JAMA* 250, no. 14 (1983): 1893–4.

12 D. J. West, G. B. Calandra, and R. W. Ellis, "Vaccination of Infants and Children Against Hepatitis B," *Pediatric Clinics of North America* 37, no. 3 (1990): 585–601. See *JAMA* 263, no. 9 (1990): 1218–22. *JAMA* 247, no. 9 (1982): 1238, reports on the impact of immigrants from Asia on the incidence in California. See also *New England Journal of Medicine* 321, no. 19 (1989): 1301–5.

13 Approximately one percent of infected adults develop acute fulminant hepatitis, which results in the rapid development of jaundice and hepatic coma; it eventually can cause brain dysfunction and death.

14 W. S. Robinson, "Hepatitis B Virus and Hepatitis Delta Virus," pp. 1214–17. See also *New England Journal of Medicine* 312, no. 5 (1985): 270–6. M. R. Hilleman, "Plasma-Derived Hepatitis B Vaccine: A Breakthrough in Preventive Medicine," in Ronald W. Ellis, ed., *Hepatitis B Vaccines in Clinical Practice* (New York, 1993), pp. 17–39. *Recombivax HB*, section 2, pp. 23, 26, MA.

HBV is the second leading, known human carcinogen, trailing only tobacco.[15]

Despite the importance of hepatitis, it was the 1940s before researchers began to achieve an understanding of the virus and the infections it caused. Some of the early work was associated with blood banks, which had a strong and direct interest in finding ways to test for the presence of HBV. Finally in the 1960s, geneticist Dr. Baruch S. Blumberg and his coworkers found that the blood from a hemophiliac reacted with the antigen in the blood of an Australian aborigine.[16] Later, after Blumberg and Dr. Alfred Prince were able to establish the relationship between the Australian antigen and HBV, scientists could use serological testing to identify hepatitis B carriers.[17] Now too they

---

15 M. R. Hilleman, "Vaccines Against Viral Hepatitis," *International Review of the Army, Navy, and Air Force Medical Services* 57, no. 1 (1984): 11–24. Each year in the United States, an estimated 4,000 people die of hepatitis B-related cirrhosis and more than 800 die from hepatitis B-related liver cancer. Worldwide, approximately 80 percent of hepatocarcinomas are caused by hepatitis B. P. Maupas and J. L. Melnick, "Hepatitis B Infection and Primary Liver Cancer," *Progress in Medical Virology* 27 (1981): 1–5. See also *New England Journal of Medicine* 305, no. 18 (1981): 1067–73.

16 B. S. Blumberg, H. J. Alter, and S. Visnich, "A 'New' Antigen in Leukemia Sera," *JAMA* 191, no. 7 (1965): 101–6. The antigen was later identified as HBsAg, a major outer-surface antigen of the virus.

17 B. S. Blumberg, B. J. S. Gerstley, D. A. Hungerford, W. T. London, and A. I. Sutnick, "A Serum Antigen (Australian Antigen) in Down's Syndrome, Leukemia, and Hepatitis," *Annals of Internal Medicine* 66, no. 5 (1967): 924–31. A. M. Prince, "An Antigen Detected in the Blood During the Incubation Period of Serum Hepatitis," *Proceedings of the National Academy of Science* 60 (1968): 814–21. *Science* 165 (July 18, 1969): 304–6. Alfred Prince at the New York Blood Center independently discovered an antigen (SH, for serum hepatitis, antigen) in persons with serum hepatitis. *Science* 170 (Oct. 16, 1970): 332–3; 176 (June 16, 1972): 1225–6. On the discussions between Blumberg (and his colleague Irving Millman) and Merck over patent rights see I. Millman, "The Development of the Hepatitis B Vaccine," in Irving Millman, Toby K. Eisenstein, and Baruch S. Blumberg, eds., *Hepatitis B: The Virus, the Disease, and the Vaccine* (New York, 1984), pp. 137–47.

could see the possibility of developing a vaccine against the disease, especially after D. S. Dane, et al. (of the Bland-Sutton Institute in London), identified the complete virus that caused hepatitis B infection. [18] HBV – thereafter also known as the "Dane particle" – is structurally, antigenically, and biologically distinct from all other known virus families. It has a long incubation period (somewhere between 40 and 180 days), and the acute disease slowly manifests itself over a period of several months. [19]

Before the development of vaccines against hepatitis, some success was achieved by administering immune serum globulin. The first effective use of immunoglobulin (with hepatitis A) was reported in 1944, and in subsequent years, some limited progress was made in establishing passive immunity against hepatitis B. [20] At Merck the research teams developed an immune globulin (*HEP-B-GAMMAGEE*, licensed in 1978) that could prevent newborn

---

18 W. S. Robinson, "Hepatitis B Virus and Hepatitis Delta Virus," pp. 1204–5. The antigen that Blumberg and Prince had independently discovered turned out to be a surface component (HBsAg) from the HBV virion.

19 T. H. Maugh II, "Hepatitis B Vaccine Passes First Major Test," *Science* 210 (Nov. 14, 1980): 760–2. Hilleman, "Vaccines Against Viral Hepatitis," pp. 11–24. W. S. Robinson, "Hepatitis B Virus and Hepatitis Delta Virus," pp. 1204–31. M. R. Hilleman, "The Vaccine Solution to the Problem of Human Hepatitis B and Its Sequelae," in R. G. Douglas, ed., *Assessment and Management of Risks Associated with Hepatitis-B: Effectiveness of Intervention* (Philadelphia, 1990), pp. 191–204. HBV is a double-shelled DNA virus belonging to the hepadnaviridae family. The virus, or "Dane particle," has a core with an outer membrane coat that drifts free when produced in excess by infected cells. The excess antigen (HBsAg) is spherical or tubular in structure and is a liposome consisting of a core of phospholipid into which surface antigen is partially embedded. By contrast with HBV, the hepatitis A virus (an RNA virus) has a relatively short incubation period of two to six weeks.

20 J. S. Mirick, R. Ward, and R. W. McCollum, "Modification of Post-Transfusion Hepatitis by Gamma Globulin," *New England Journal of Medicine* 273, no. 2 (1965): 59–65.

---

infants of carrier mothers from becoming HBV carriers themselves. The new immune globulin was also useful with nonimmune individuals who have had a relatively low-volume exposure, such as an accidental needle stick.[21]

Virus and Cell Biology's major goal, however, was to develop an effective vaccine for hepatitis B. Because the virus could not be cultivated in cell culture, the vaccine research could not follow the path established with the polio, measles, mumps, and rubella vaccines. Building on the discoveries by Prince and Blumberg, Hilleman and his crew set out to chart a new course in 1968, first by purifying the antigen and developing assay procedures.[22] Their working hypothesis was that antibody developed against the surface antigen (HBsAg) would afford protection against the virus. If that was the case and if they could obtain sufficient amounts of HBsAg from the blood plasma of persons who were carriers, they thought they could produce a vaccine.[23] In addition to being purified, the antigen would have to be inactivated and rendered free of infectivity from all life-forms potentially present in human blood – without losing its immunizing potency.

---

21 Hilleman, "Plasma-Derived Hepatitis B Vaccine: A Breakthrough in Preventive Medicine," p. 17. *Recombivax HB*, section 2, pp. 31–2, MA. Later, the immune globulin was administered in conjunction with a hepatitis B vaccine to provide immediate protection until the vaccine stimulated an active and long-lasting immune response. Protection conferred by immune globulin is only of short-term duration, however, and is ineffective in cases of high-level virus exposure such as occurs in a transfusion with infected blood. See also *Pediatrics* 72, no. 2 (1983): 176–80.

22 The major team members included William J. McAleer, Alfred A. Tytell, Eugene B. Buynak, George P. Lampson, and Robert R. Roehm. Hilleman had begun to discuss a possible hepatitis vaccine with Tishler in 1960. M. R. Hilleman to M. Tishler, July 5, 1960, MA.

23 As of 1969, Hilleman was not publicly optimistic about the possibilities of producing a hepatitis vaccine. See M. R. Hilleman, "Toward Control of Viral Infections of Man," *Science* 164 (May 2, 1969): 509.

Even in the days before AIDS was discovered, purification and inactivation were crucial steps in the process of vaccine development.[24] Merck's researchers initially tried two approaches to inactivation, one physical-chemical, and the other entirely chemical. MSDRL's Rahway instrument labs developed a new piece of equipment that ran physically purified virus through an ultraviolet irradiation tube and then through a heat exchange pipe (hot oil bath), before treating it with formaldehyde. But Hilleman's teams chose the competing chemical approach, which applied three virus-killing procedures;[25] it yielded antigen that was nearly 100 percent pure.[26]

As yet, however, they did not have any assurance that they could recover enough antigen to make the vaccine a realistic innovation. Dr. Saul Krugman, professor of pediatrics at New York University College of Medicine, helped Hilleman and his colleagues solve that problem. Krugman was to hepatitis what Robert Austrian was to pneumonia. Through the 1960s, Krugman and his coworkers had been studying hepatitis in human subjects in the Willowbrook School in New York.[27] In the course of their experiments, they explored ways to

---

24 See the comments in M. R. Hilleman, A. U. Bertland, E. B. Buynak, G. P. Lampson, W. J. McAleer, A. A. McLean, R. R. Roehm, and A. A. Tytell, "Clinical and Laboratory Studies of HBsAg Vaccine," in Girish N. Vyas, Stephen N. Cohen, and Rudi Schmid, eds., *Viral Hepatitis: A Contemporary Assessment of Etiology, Epidemiology, Pathogenesis and Prevention* (Philadelphia, 1978), pp. 525–7. As the authors note, "there is no in vitro means to detect residual live virus."

25 The solely chemical procedure won out because of the purity of the antigen it produced and because it could be relied on to destroy human scrapie-like infectious material that might cause Creutzfeld-Jakob syndrome if present in sufficient amount. On the latter syndrome see J. R. Lehrich and K. L. Tyler, "Slow Infections of the Central Nervous System," in Mandell, Douglas, and Bennett, eds., *Infectious Diseases*, p. 772.

26 M. R. Hilleman, "Notes," MA.

27 J. J. Lander, J. P. Giles, R. H. Purcell, and S. Krugman, "Viral Hepatitis, Type B (MS-2 Strain)," *New England Journal of Medicine* 285, no. 6 (1971): 303–7. *JAMA* 220, no. 7 (1972): 908–9.

inactivate HBV in human blood products.[28] Their 1971 report provided a clue to the problem that was worrying Hilleman, who obtained a sample of Krugman's boiled plasma. He discovered that it contained enough antigen to make the vaccine project feasible.[29]

By 1975 Merck was prepared to start clinical testing in human subjects, but Hilleman foresaw serious problems.[30] The first tests had to be done where there was least chance for natural exposure to hepatitis B, since an inadvertent coinfection might undermine the company's

28 Krugman, et al., diluted human carrier serum 1/10 and exposed it to boiling temperature in sealed glass containers for one minute. As they discovered, most but not all the virus was destroyed. To assay for retained infectivity, Krugman injected the preparation into human subjects and was surprised to note that the material was able to stimulate specific hepatitis B surface antigen antibody. Some of the subjects also developed core antibody, indicating incomplete inactivation. Krugman next discovered that most of his subjects had as a result of the experiment acquired substantial protection from the disease. See Krugman's commentary on this experiment in L. Bianchi, W. Gerok, K. Sickinger, and G. A. Stalder, eds., *Virus and the Liver*, Falk Symposium 28 (Lancaster, 1980), pp. 387–9; and Hilleman's additions, pp. 389–94. See also E. B. Buynak, R. R. Roehm, A. A. Tytell, A. U. Bertland, G. P. Lampson, and M. R. Hilleman, "Vaccine Against Human Hepatitis B," *JAMA* 235, no. 26 (1976): 2832–4.

29 S. Krugman, J. P. Giles, and J. Hammond, "Viral Hepatitis, Type B (MS-2 Strain): Studies on Active Immunization," *JAMA* 217, no. 1 (1971): 41–5. M. R. Hilleman, "Immunologic Prevention of Human Hepatitis," *Perspectives in Biology and Medicine* 27, no. 4 (1984): 543–57. Hilleman, "Plasma-Derived Hepatitis B Vaccine: A Breakthrough in Preventive Medicine," pp. 17–39.

30 E. B. Buynak, R. R. Roehm, A. A. Tytell, A. U. Bertland, G. P. Lampson, and M. R. Hilleman, "Development and Chimpanzee Testing of a Vaccine Against Human Hepatitis B," *Proceedings of the Society for Experimental Biology and Medicine* 151 (1976): 694-700. M. R. Hilleman, E. B. Buynak, R. R. Roehm, A. A. Tytell, A. U. Bertland, and G. P. Lampson, "Purified and Inactivated Human Hepatitis B Vaccine: Progress Report," *American Journal of the Medical Sciences* 270, no. 2 (1975): 401–4. Buynak, Roehm, Tytell, Bertland, Lampson, and Hilleman, "Vaccine Against Human Hepatitis B," pp. 2832–4. Merck added alum adjuvant to increase the immunizing potency of the vaccine prepared for clinical trial.

Edward M. Scolnick,
M.D., President of
Merck Research
Laboratories.

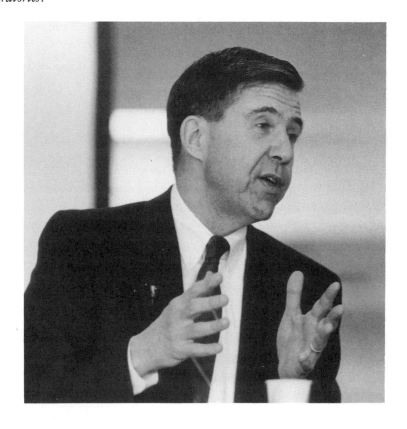

support for the new product. The safest place for the initial tests seemed to be inside Merck. Since the lab personnel in Virus and Cell Biology (including Hilleman) had been exposed, they recruited a group of volunteers from the company's high supervisory levels. Saul Krugman gave the first injections (to himself, his wife, and nine Merck supervisory personnel), and six months later, there were no indications of infection in any of the volunteers.

After working out an optimal regime for immunization, Merck

arranged for a more extensive clinical trial.[31] This was conducted by Dr. Wolf Szmuness, head of epidemiology for the New York Blood Center. For several years, Szmuness had been conducting epidemiologic studies of hepatitis B in New York City's gay population – a group particularly susceptible to the disease. He now agreed to run a two-year trial (launched in 1978, under double-blind control) among homosexual males. Half received vaccine and half placebo.[32] By 1980, the results were in. One hundred percent of the men who had responded serologically to the vaccine were protected against hepatitis B, while the infection continued unabated in the control group.[33] Additional trials yielded similar results.[34] The DBS promptly (November 1981) granted

31 By 1978, Virus and Cell Biology had settled on the following regime: two initial doses of vaccine given a month apart, followed by a booster five months later. This afforded the best chance for achieving a rapid initial immunity and for expanding the memory cell bank by the booster, thus providing long-lasting immunity.

32 Dr. Cladd E. Stevens, who had studied hepatitis B epidemiology in Taiwan, assisted Szmuness. Dr. Saul Krugman, Dr. Robert McCollum (Yale), and Hilleman comprised the informed monitoring group.

33 W. Szmuness, C. E. Stevens, E. J. Harley, E. A. Zang, W. R. Oleszko, D. C. William, R. Sadovsky, J. M. Morrison, and A. Kellner, "Hepatitis B Vaccine: Demonstration of Efficacy in a Controlled Clinical Trial in a High-Risk Population in the United States," *New England Journal of Medicine* 303, no. 15 (1980): 833–41; see also the editorial comment on pp. 874–6; and the discussion in 304, no. 6 (1981): 363–4. See also *Nature* 287 (Oct. 9, 1980): 483–4.

34 Dr. James Maynard and Dr. Donald Francis, then at the CDC hepatitis unit in Phoenix, Arizona, conducted a second, confirmatory study, also among gay men. As subsequent studies indicated, immunosuppressed and immunoincompetent individuals, as well as the mentally retarded, showed a slow or reduced response. The most powerful indicator of response to the vaccine in normal people was age. The elderly exhibited a slower response and a degree of reduction in seroconversion. But since the vaccine was most needed in young people and children, who responded extremely well, this was not thought to be a serious problem. Maugh, "Hepatitis B Vaccine Passes First Major Test," pp. 760–2. M. R. Hilleman, E. B. Buynak, W. J. McAleer, and A. A. McLean, "Human Hepatitis B Vaccine," in Saul Krugman and S. Sherlock, eds., *Proceedings of the European Symposium on Hepatitis B* (New York, 1981), pp. 120–39. Krugman,

Merck a license to produce and market *Heptavax-B*, the first subunit viral vaccine produced in the United States.[35]

The company had already begun large-scale production in anticipation of government licensing. Merck, which had recently invested $8 million in upgrading its vaccine production facilities, was able through process innovation to triple the antigen recovery rate. This innovation and the lead time were important because the complex manufacturing process took sixty-five weeks — the longest production time of any vaccine then being manufactured.[36] Nevertheless, the firm

---

"The Newly Licensed Hepatitis B Vaccine," pp. 2012–15; also *JAMA* 250, no. 1 (1983): 19; and 258, no. 9 (1987): 1193–5. Hilleman, "Plasma-Derived Hepatitis B Vaccine," pp. 17–39. *New England Journal of Medicine* 307, no. 24 (1982): 1481–6; 311, no. 8 (1984): 496–501; 315, no. 4 (1986): 209–14; 321, no. 11 (1989): 708–12. *Lancet* (Nov. 26, 1983): 1245; (Dec. 24/31, 1983): 1454–6; (Oct. 13, 1984): 866; (Oct. 27, 1984): 983; (June 22, 1985): 1412–15; (Oct. 7, 1989): 847–9. *Pediatrics* 83, no. 6 (1989): 1041–8.

35 Krugman, "The Newly Licensed Hepatitis B Vaccine," pp. 2012–15. Hilleman, "Vaccines Against Viral Hepatitis," pp. 11–24. Hilleman, "Plasma-Derived Hepatitis B Vaccine," pp. 17–39. M. R. Hilleman, Interview, Nov. 13 and 21, 1991. The Pasteur Institute began marketing a hepatitis B vaccine at approximately this same time. Millman, "The Development of the Hepatitis B Vaccine," p. 137. See also the report on the subsequent CDC clinical trial in *Annals of Internal Medicine* 97, no. 3 (1982): 362–6; and M. R. Hilleman, W. J. McAleer, E. B. Buynak, and A. A. McLean, "Quality and Safety of Human Hepatitis B Vaccine," *Developments in Biological Standardization* 54 (1983): 3–12. *Lancet* (Dec. 3, 1983): 1301; see *Lancet* (Dec. 10, 1983): 1323–8 for a report on a clinical trial of a vaccine prepared by the Netherlands Red Cross Blood Transfusion Service.

36 As Hilleman later observed, "Technologically, development of the vaccine was the most difficult challenge we have ever faced. We had to develop entirely new methods of vaccine preparation, create new measurement criteria and techniques for the production cycle, and develop sophisticated new testing methods." Less formally, he characterized it as "a small nightmare in a sea of ignorance." M. R. Hilleman, "Notes"; and Press release, Nov. 16, 1981; both in MA. Hilleman, McAleer, Buynak, and McLean, "Quality and Safety of Human Hepatitis B Vaccine," pp. 3–12.

---

announced (November 1981) that *Heptavax-B* would be available by mid-1982 in sufficient quantities to meet the needs of the entire country. By July 1982, the new production facilities had achieved that goal.[37] The vaccine they produced was recommended for infants, children, and adults who were at high risk of contracting hepatitis B infection.[38]

After thirteen years of research, development, and production, Merck's biological group had produced a new vaccine that would in the years ahead provide protection from HBV for more than 1.5 million people.[39] That figure would have been much larger, however, had the vaccine been less difficult and costly to make. When Hilleman and his coworkers were completing their efforts on *Heptavax-B*, they already knew that they "could never make enough vaccine to handle the market." It was simply too difficult to locate an adequate supply of suitable carrier plasma.[40] Even when they did, the vaccine was very expensive to manufacture and test. At that time, it was the most expensive ever produced and was sold at $100 for the three doses needed to immunize.

---

37 R. Frank Ecock, Interview, Nov. 4, 1991.

38 *JAMA* 246, no. 19 (1981): 2111–12. Krugman, "The Newly Licensed Hepatitis B Vaccine," pp. 2014–15; and *JAMA* 247, no. 16 (1982): 2272–6. See also R. E. Weibel, "Hepatitis B Vaccine Trials, Experience and Review," in Millman, Eisenstein, and Blumberg, eds., *Hepatitis B*, pp. 161–74. See also *Journal of the American Geriatric Society* 30, no. 5 (1982): 326–8; *Military Medicine* 147, no. 6 (1982): 506–8; and *Pediatric Infectious Disease Journal* 1, no. 4 (1982): 217–18; and 2, no. 4 (1983): 273–5. *New England Journal of Medicine* 308, no. 5 (1983): 280–1; and 311, no. 10 (1984): 684–8. *Pediatrics* 71, no. 2 (1983): 289–92.

39 *Pediatrics* 75, no. 2 (1985): 362–4.

40 See the discussion in S. Funakoshi, T. Ohmura, T. Fujiwara, T. Suyama, and R. Naito, "Large-Scale Production of Hepatitis B Vaccine," *Progress in Medical Virology* 27 (1981): 163–7. The Green Cross Corporation, Osaka, Japan, had prepared its first lot of hepatitis B vaccine. See also *Nature* 290 (Mar. 5, 1981): 51–4.

This precluded use in many of the countries where the vaccine was most needed.[41]

There were, as well, widespread concerns in the early 1980s about any plasma-based product. In 1981, scientists first recognized the acquired immunodeficiency syndrome (AIDS), spreading fear that Merck's new vaccine and others might be contaminated. It was, after all, 1983 before the causal virus (HIV) was even isolated. Subsequently, Merck established that its decontamination procedures killed any HIV in the plasma, but meanwhile the introduction of the new vaccine was slowed.[42] While widespread administration of the vaccine seemed to be called for, many insurance companies in the United States

---

41 D. P. Francis, "Elective Primary Health Care: Strategies for Control of Disease in the Developing World. III. Hepatitis B Virus and Its Related Diseases," *Reviews of Infectious Diseases* 5, no. 2 (1983): 322–9. M. Kane, "The Task of Epidemiology in Designing Strategies for the Use of Hepatitis B Vaccine," *Public Health Reports* 99, no. 3 (1984): 264–6.

But also see cost-benefit analyses in *Lancet* (Aug. 22, 1987): 441–2; in *New England Journal of Medicine* 307, no. 11 (1982): 644–52, 678–9; 308, no. 2 (1983): 104–5; and *JAMA* 250, no. 16 (1983): 2145–50; 251, no. 21 (1984): 2765–7, 2771; 251, no. 21 (1984): 2794. "To state it simply," Hilleman later observed, "the vaccine for the most part sits on the shelf." Hilleman, "Plasma-Derived Hepatitis B Vaccine," p. 32. See also the discussion in *Lancet* (Aug. 18, 1984): 405–6; and *Lancet* (Nov. 10, 1984): 1091–2; *Nature* 312 (Nov. 15, 1984): 190; and Hilleman's reply in 313 (Jan. 17, 1985): 176; see also 317 (Oct. 30, 1985): 489–95.

42 D. P. Francis, P. M. Feorino, S. McDougal, D. Warfield, J. Getchell, C. Cabradilla, M. Tong, W. J. Miller, L. D. Schultz, F. J. Bailey, W. J. McAleer, E. M. Scolnick, and R. W. Ellis, "The Safety of the Hepatitis B Vaccine: Inactivation of the AIDS Virus During Routine Vaccine Manufacture," *JAMA* 256, no. 7 (1986): 869–72. See also *JAMA* 249, no. 6 (1983): 685–6, 745–6; 249, no. 14 (1983): 1812; 250, no. 14 (1983): 1891–2; 252, no. 24 (1984): 3375–7; 253, no. 1 (1985): 21; 254, no. 8 (1985): 1064–6; 255, no. 6 (1986): 716; *New England Journal of Medicine* 308, no. 19 (1983): 1163–4; 311, no. 16 (1984): 1030–2; 312 (1985): 375-6; 315, no. 4 (1986): 250–2; *Nature* 304, no. 14 (1983): 104; and 304, no. 28 (1983): 297; *Pediatrics* 72, no. 2 (1983): 265–6; *Lancet* (June 29, 1985): 1506–7; *American Journal of Public Health* 76, no. 3 (1986): 252–5; 78, no. 8 (1988): 973–4.

refused to pay for *Heptavax-B*.[43] Merck was left with an uphill battle that did not bode well for the new product.

2

Merck's efforts to solve these problems by developing an alternative hepatitis B vaccine carried Virus and Cell Biology into a new long cycle of scientific and technical discovery. There were new networks to tend outside the firm, and within the organization, a new cadre of leaders. There were, in brief, abundant opportunities for the company's vaccine operations to falter and perhaps to fail completely in making this demanding transition.

Hilleman's team began the search for a less expensive vaccine from sources other than plasma by examining Alexander cells as a means of producing antigen. The Alexander cells are a line of liver cancer cells derived from an HBV carrier. Because it is a cancer cell, it grows continuously in cell culture and because it bears the integrated genetic sequence of hepatitis B virus, it sheds hepatitis B surface antigen. Using specially designed culture techniques, the Merck team coaxed the Alexander cells to produce the antigen in quantities that would make the production process economically comparable to the plasma-derived antigen. They produced in vitro a vaccine that was as potent as *Heptavax-B*, and the initial tests in animals and human cancer patients indicated that it was well tolerated and efficacious.[44]

---

43 Krugman, "The Newly Licensed Hepatitis B Vaccine," pp. 2012–15. *New York Times*, Dec. 16, 1984. Hilleman, "The Vaccine Solution to the Problem of Human Hepatitis B and Its Sequelae," pp. 191–204. In Belgium, as of 1983, health insurance covered the cost of the vaccine. *Lancet* (Oct. 17, 1987): 913.

44 W. J. McAleer, H. Z. Markus, F. J. Bailey, A. C. Herman, B. J. Harder, D. E. Wampler, W. J. Miller, P. M. Keller, E. B. Buynak, and M. R. Hilleman, "Production of Purified Hepatitis B Surface Antigen from Alexander Hepatoma Cells Grown in Artificial Capillary Units," *Journal of Virological Methods* 7, nos. 5–6 (1983): 263–71. W. J. McAleer, H. Z. Markus, E. E. Wampler, E. B. Buynak, W. J. Miller, R. E. Weibel, A. A. McLean, and M. R. Hilleman, "Vaccine Against Human Hepatitis B Virus Prepared from Antigen Derived from Human Hepatoma Cells in Culture," *Proceedings of the Society for Experimental*

But the company decided not to continue down this path. Because the laboratory was deriving the antigen from a cancer cell, the product would raise questions about the safety of normal children being immunized. Even when the firm had demonstrated that the AIDS virus could not survive in *Heptavax-B*, there had been resistance to vaccination with the product. Although the company's scientists already had procedures to assure safety by purifying and inactivating residual nucleic acid in the new vaccine, the product was likely to remain suspect in the relevant networks.[45]

Besides, several years before, Roy Vagelos had seen a different route toward a safe and less expensive hepatitis B vaccine. New developments in DNA technology and in molecular biology were making it possible for researchers to use fragments of DNA to produce specific antigens in microbial cells. As the transformed cells divided, they replicated the antigens. Seeing the potential of recombinant DNA technology, Vagelos set out to convince the Virus and Cell Biology research team to explore this new area of science simultaneously with the work they were doing with Alexander cells.[46] He brought microbi-

Biology and Medicine 175 (1984): 314–19. The Merck teams developed an artificial, vitafiber, capillary system for growing the Alexander cells.

45 M. R. Hilleman, E. B. Buynak, H. Z. Markus, R. Z. Maigetter, W. J. McAleer, A. A. McLean, W. J. Miller, D. E. Wampler, and R. E. Weibel, "Control of Hepatitis B Virus Infection: Vaccines Produced from Alexander Cell Line and from Recombinant Yeast Cell Cultures," in Girish N. Vyas, Jules L. Dienstag, and Jay H. Hoofnagle, eds., *Viral Hepatitis and Liver Disease* (Orlando, FL, 1984), p. 313, explains that: "The most important advantages of the recombinant vaccine relate to simpler HBsAg production by yeast cells in fermentation tanks and removal of any lingering apprehensions about safety of vaccine derived from a human cancer cell source."

46 Researchers at the National Institute of Allergy and Infectious Diseases had developed a genetically altered influenza virus vaccine. *JAMA* 221, no. 11 (1972): 1217–18. See also *Virology* 78 (1977): 183–91; 83 (1977): 356–64; 88 (1978): 231–43, 244–51; R. A. Lerner, "Synthetic Vaccines," *Scientific American* 248 (Feb. 1983): 66–74; and *Nature* 311 (Sept. 6, 1984): 12–13, 67–9; 311 (Oct. 11, 1984): 578–9.

ologist Jerome Birnbaum into the discussions in order to achieve this objective. In this instance – as in the previous move into bacterial vaccines – the autonomy of Virus and Cell Biology's process of innovation was qualified in a significant way. Without having done so, Merck might well have been on the sidelines during the next long cycle in vaccine innovation.

Vagelos used Birnbaum as the interface between Virus and Cell Biology and Dr. William Rutter, an eminent molecular biochemist at the University of California. They worked out a collaborative research program for a recombinant expression system to produce hepatitis B antigen in microbial cells. Cloning or genetic engineering by way of recombinant DNA technology had begun at the end of the 1960s and by the early 1970s had already produced its first technical breakthroughs. Using this novel technique, researchers were able to insert new genetic information (e.g., that of hepatitis B surface antigen) into a plasmid, a circular piece of self-replicating episomal DNA normally present in a microbial cell, and to cause expression of the added genetic information. This novel technique was patented and termed "genetic splicing."

The goal was to produce the antigen Merck needed in microbes. The scientific reasoning was impeccable, but the goal proved elusive. Dr. Pablo Valenzuela, working in Rutter's laboratory, undertook the gene splicing, and after two years of work, he succeeded in expressing HBsAg in the bacterium *E. coli*.[47] Although Valenzuela was

---

47 P. Valenzuela, P. Gray, M. Quiroga, J. Zaldivar, H. M. Goodman, and W. J. Rutter, "Nucleotide Sequence of the Gene Coding for the Major Protein of Hepatitis B Virus Surface Antigen," *Nature* 280 (Aug. 30, 1979): 815–19. See also C. J. Burrell, P. Mackay, P. J. Greenaway, P. H. Hofschneider, and K. Murray, "Expression in *Escherichia Coli* of Hepatitis B Virus DNA Sequences Cloned in Plasmid pBR322," *Nature* 279 (May 3, 1970): 43–7; and J. C. Edman, R. A. Hallewell, P. Valenzuela, H. M. Goodman, and W. J. Rutter, "Synthesis of Hepatitis B Surface and Core Antigens in *E. Coli*," *Nature* 291 (June 11, 1981): 503–6.

now able to produce the correct antigen (226 amino acid S polypeptide), his subunit of the virus would not prompt the immunologic response Merck needed. This form of HBsAg, they learned, did not assume a conformational folding characteristic of the natural antigen and essential to its specificity.[48]

About the time that these disappointing results came in, however, MSDRL learned that a new path had been opened to a recombinant antigen. Both Genentech, one of the country's leading biotech companies, and Dr. Benjamin D. Hall of the University of Washington had discovered plasmids (i.e., episomal units) in ordinary bakers' yeast.[49] Yeast, like human cells, is a eukaryote that might provide for more natural folding of HBsAg, and Merck decided to explore this approach. In addition, yeast could be grown *en masse* in fermentation tanks, an important consideration if the company was going to reduce the cost of its vaccine significantly.

Merck quickly worked out a quadripartite, cooperative program among Merck's Virus and Cell Biology, Rutter's team at the University of California, Hall's laboratory at the University of Washington, and the Chiron Corporation, a California biotech firm.[50] Their joint efforts produced vectors that carried the DNA sequence of the hepatitis B antigen. By transferring the vectors to yeast (*Saccharomyces cerevisiae*), they were able to produce an antigen that folded in the same manner as natural HBsAg, that formed the typical liposomal particles

---

48 Ibid. M. R. Hilleman, "Notes," MA. See also *Nature* 295 (Jan. 14, 1982): 158–60.

49 On Genentech see Robert Teitelman, *Gene Dreams: Wall Street, Academia, and the Rise of Biotechnology* (New York, 1989); and the same author's *Profits of Science: The American Marriage of Business and Technology* (New York, 1994). P. Valenzuela, A. Medina, W. J. Rutter, G. Ammerer, and B. D. Hall, "Synthesis and Assembly of Hepatitis B Virus Surface Antigen Particles in Yeast," *Nature* 298 (July 22, 1982): 347–50.

50 On Chiron see Teitelman, *Gene Dreams*, pp. 138, 198; and Shawn L. Linam and M. Todd Jarvis, *Biotechnology Sourcebook* (Madison, GA, 1989), pp. 86–9.

of the natural antigen, and that stimulated the sought-after antibody reaction.[51]

Just as Merck seemed to be getting closer to success, the Hilleman era drew to a close and Dr. Edward M. Scolnick took over as Virus and Cell Biology's new scientific leader. Seen in retrospect, this institutional transition actually took place over several years. It had begun when Vagelos pushed the hepatitis vaccine project toward recombinant DNA technology and went outside the firm to obtain the new scientific capabilities Merck needed in biotechnology. At that point, Merck did not yet have the in-house scientific resources and personnel it needed to move into this new field. Vagelos also went outside the firm to recruit Scolnick, whose background in biosynthesis and genetic research made him an ideal science leader to develop the new capabilities the company needed.

One of Scolnick's first jobs was to convince his colleagues that the new cycle taking shape was bringing a fundamental, formative restructuring of the process of innovation in biomedical science. "It was the transistor," he said, "and not just a better light bulb!" As a distinguished research scientist, he was concerned to find that his new

---

51 Valenzuela, Medina, Rutter, Ammerer, and Hall, "Synthesis and Assembly of Hepatitis B Virus Surface Antigen Particles in Yeast," pp. 347–50. W. J. Mc-Aleer, E. B. Buynak, R. Z. Maigetter, D. E. Wampler, W. J. Miller, and M. R. Hilleman, "Human Hepatitis B Vaccine from Recombinant Yeast," *Nature* 307 (Jan. 12, 1984): 178–80. As Hilleman noted: "The S antigen gene of the viral DNA was excised from the double-stranded viral DNA, flanked by promoter and terminator sequences, and inserted into the ring structure of the plasmid vector. . . . Transfected into yeast, this plasmid faithfully encodes for production of surface antigen polypeptide that then can be readily purified from the yeast cell lysate." M. R. Hilleman, "Vaccine Perspectives from the Vantage of Hepatitis B," *Vaccine Research* 1, no. 1 (1992): 6. See also A. J. Zuckerman, "Developing Synthetic Vaccines," *Nature* 295 (Jan. 14, 1982): 98–9; and 296 (Apr. 29, 1982): 792, on a recombinant DNA veterinary vaccine produced by Intervet International, a Dutch firm. On Genentech's similar work see *Nucleic Acids Research* 11, no. 9 (1983): 2745–63.

Dr. David Krah of the Merck Research Laboratories discusses a computer picture of the varicella (chicken pox) virus.

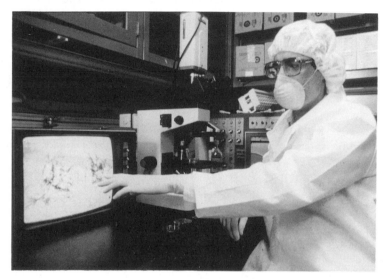

organization was from his perspective several years behind the front edge of the field. He set out to accelerate the transition, focusing at first on the hepatitis B vaccine that Merck was now working on with Chiron.[52]

First as executive director (1982) and then as a vice president (1983) in charge of Virus and Cell Biology Research, Scolnick and his team took over the research on the new vaccine. Much remained to be

---

52 Interview, Edward M. Scolnick, July 17, 1995. As Dr. Stephen Drew, who was lead process engineer on the project, later commented: "It was clear right away that Scolnick brought a focus and perspective that transcended the existing organization." Interview, Aug. 30, 1995. The focus was now on the molecular mechanisms.

done with the vectors received from the Chiron Corporation.[53] In an effort to accelerate that work, Scolnick pulled some of his best researchers off a cancer project (his strongest research interest prior to joining Merck) and used them in the complex research and development process. He also brought in new scientific personnel, including a specialist in yeast genetics.[54] While Scolnick guided Virus and Cell Biology toward a better understanding of the new science, experienced researchers like William McAleer helped their new leader master the practical aspects of vaccine development.[55]

There was much to be done to realize the potential of this breakthrough in biotechnology and genetic science.[56] The procedures

---

53 In Scolnick's view, Chiron had provided proof of the principle that the antigen could be made in yeast, but Merck did not have what it needed for large-scale production of a vaccine. Edward M. Scolnick, Interview, July 15, 1995. In order to accelerate the process of scaling up, Merck solved the problems involved concurrently (instead of sequentially). Stephen Drew, Interview, Aug. 30, 1995. Loren D. Schultz, Interview, Aug. 31, 1995.

54 The specialist in yeast genetics was Dr. Loren D. Schultz, who had done his graduate work with Dr. Benjamin Hall at the University of Washington. Schultz headed the effort to work up the vectors received from Chiron. One of the problems was that Chiron was at that time new to the process of preparing products for FDA approval. Loren D. Schultz, Interview, Aug. 31, 1995. Dr. Ronald W. Ellis, who had worked with Scolnick on cancer research at NIH, also joined the Virus and Cell Biology team. See, for instance, Ronald D. Ellis, ed., *Vaccines: New Approaches to Immunological Problems* (Boston, 1992).

55 Edward M. Scolnick, Interview, July 17, 1995. Scolnick made it clear at this time that Virus and Cell Biology was setting up a state-of-the-art laboratory in the new science/technology – a laboratory that would generalize the innovations in genetic science and DNA technology over a broad range of potential products. Loren D. Schultz, Interview, Aug. 31, 1995.

56 Virus and Cell Biology had first to discover ways to preserve the culture, then expand the production strain, and next develop the process for large-scale fermentation. Meanwhile, protein purification studies were underway. Loren D. Schultz, Interview, Aug. 31, 1995. Stephen Drew, Interview, Aug. 30, 1995.

For a different approach see G. L. Smith, M. Mackett, and B. Moss, involved fermentation of the yeast; centrifugation to separate the yeast from the broth; and rupture of the yeast cells to release the antigen, which was then separated, ultrafiltered, and purified. After treatment with formaldehyde, the purified surface antigen was used to prepare the vaccine by adsorbing it to aluminum hydroxide adjuvant and preserving it with thimerosal.[57]

Then the new teams guided the vaccine through its initial clinical tests in humans.[58] They first administered the experimental vaccine to two groups of human volunteers at Merck, and within three months, 80 to 100 percent had produced antibodies specific to HBsAg. There were no serious reactions to this test, apparently the first in history to use in humans a vaccine prepared by cloning. The level of protection was comparable with that induced by the company's plasma-based vaccine,

---

"Infectious Vaccinia Virus Recombinants That Express Hepatitis B Virus Surface Antigen," *Nature* 302 (Apr. 7, 1983): 490–5; and the comment on pp. 476–7; and in 306 (Dec. 1, 1983): 427. See also *Nature* 317 (Oct. 31, 1985): 813–15; 319 (Feb. 13, 1986): 543, 549–50.

57 M. R. Hilleman, W. J. McAleer, E. B. Buynak, A. A. McLean, P. J. Provost, and D. E. Wampler, "Future Vaccines Against Hepatitis," in S. K. Sam, C. L. Lai, and E. K. Yeo, eds., *Viral Hepatitis B Infection in the Western Pacific Region: Vaccine and Control*, Proceedings of the Western Pacific Regional Workshop on Hepatitis B, Hong Kong, Sept. 10–11, 1983 (Singapore, 1984), pp. 237–54. McAleer, Buynak, Maigetter, Wampler, Miller, and Hilleman, "Human Hepatitis B Vaccine from Recombinant Yeast," pp. 178–80. Hilleman, "Immunologic Prevention of Human Hepatitis," pp. 543–57. Hilleman, "The Vaccine Solution to the Problem of Human Hepatitis B and Its Sequelae," pp. 191–204. *Recombivax HB*, section 3, p. 5, MA.

58 The team included a number of the regulars from Hilleman's group, including Arlene A. McLean, William J. McAleer, William J. Miller, and Eugene B. Buynak. On the safety and animal tests see McAleer, Buynak, Maigetter, Wampler, Miller, and Hilleman, "Human Hepatitis B Vaccine from Recombinant Yeast," pp. 178–80; and M. R. Hilleman, R. E. Weibel, and E. M. Scolnick, "Recombinant Yeast Human Hepatitis B Vaccine," *Journal of the Hong Kong Medical Association* 37, no. 2 (1985): 75–85.

Heptavax-B.[59] Larger clinical tests confirmed these results, as did the tests in children and infants.[60] The vaccine protected the population most at risk to become HBV carriers — neonates born to mothers who are seropositive for the HBV antigen.

After these tests were successfully completed, the West German government licensed the new vaccine in May of 1986, followed in July by the United States.[61] *Recombivax HB* was the world's first vaccine for humans produced by recombinant technology.[62] By this time, the

---

59 E. M. Scolnick, A. A. McLean, D. J. West, W. J. McAleer, W. J. Miller, and E. B. Buynak, "Clinical Evaluation in Healthy Adults of a Hepatitis B Vaccine Made by Recombinant DNA," *JAMA* 251, no. 21 (1984): 2812–15; also see 258, no. 11 (1987): 1474. Merck conducted studies on antibody seroconversion in human vaccine recipients to compare the performance of the yeast- and the plasma-derived vaccines. MSDRL researchers found that the rate and rapidity of seroconversion in subjects given a ten μg. dose of the yeast vaccine was almost identical with that of subjects who received either a ten μg. or twenty μg. dose of the plasma vaccine. Of the vaccine recipients tested one month after their second dose, 87 percent had developed antibody, and following the booster dose at six months, the antibody had been stimulated in 96 to 99 percent of the subjects. See also *Lancet* (Jan. 12, 1985): 108–9; and *Lancet* (Feb. 23, 1985): 455–6.

60 Hilleman, Weibel, and Scolnick, "Recombinant Yeast Human Hepatitis B Vaccine," pp. 75–85. M. R. Hilleman, "Hepatitis B and AIDS and the Promise for Their Control by Vaccines," *Vaccine* 6 (Apr. 1988): 175–9. M. R. Hilleman, "Vaccine Perspectives from the Vantage of Hepatitis B," pp. 11–13. See also *JAMA* 253, no. 12 (1985): 1740–5; 261, no. 16 (1989): 2362–6. *Lancet* (Sept. 26, 1987): 728–31.

61 Scolnick recentralized the vaccine clinical operations, moving them back into MSD's clinical research organization. This institutional change was part of Scolnick's general strategy of making Virus and Cell Biology less self-contained; the transition was facilitated by the improvements Vagelos had promoted in MSD clinical research.

62 In September 1989, the Food and Drug Administration would approve Engerix-B, SmithKline Beecham's new recombinant DNA vaccine against hepatitis B virus infections. SmithKline Beecham, Press Release, Sept. 8, 1989, MA. See also *JAMA* 261, no. 22 (1989): 3278–81. SmithKline Beecham announced that it would sell three doses of its vaccine for the average wholesale price of

---

company's effort to catch up in genetic research and recombinant DNA technology was succeeding. This placed Merck in a strategic position in a rapidly evolving science-technology network that was beginning to generate a broad range of important opportunities for vaccine innovation.[63] The new recombinant vaccine would also open the way for a global campaign against hepatitis B, a campaign that might someday have the same impact on this disease that vaccination had already had on smallpox.[64]

3

Recombivax HB gave Merck a significant role to play in the international campaigns then underway to improve immunization rates in the developing nations. The World Health Organization (WHO), the United Nations, and the Pan American Health Organization (PAHO) were the leading institutions mobilizing resources to combat disease in the developing countries where neither governments nor individuals could usually afford vaccines.[65] In 1967 WHO had led a multinational, cooperative program for smallpox eradication and within a

---

$149.20, undercutting Merck's average wholesale price of $170.51 (also for three doses) of *Recombivax HB*. The Belgian government had approved the SmithKline vaccine in 1986. *Nature* 324 (Dec. 11, 1986): 506. *World Health Organization Drug Information* 1, no. 2 (1987): 67. This resulting competition was expressed in part through a battle of the clinical studies. *JAMA* 259, no. 16 (1988): 2402–4. *Pediatric Infectious Disease Journal* 10, no. 4 (1991): 299–303.

Japan's Chemo-Sero-Therapeutic Research Institute (Kaketsuken) also entered the competition. *Nature* 337 (January 12, 1989): 106.

63 See, for instance, *Nature* 311 (Oct. 11, 1984): 510-11; 312 (Nov. 22, 1984): 299; 335 (Sept. 15, 1988): 259–62.

64 But even with the recombinant vaccine available, safety concerns could still influence decisions about immunization. *American Journal of Public Health* 79, no. 1 (1989): 101–2.

65 On the scientific activities of WHO see, for instance, World Health Organization, "Human Viral and Rickettsial Vaccines," *World Health Organization Technical Report Series* 325 (1966). World Health Organization, *Sixth Report on the World Health Situation, 1973–1977*, part 1, *Global Analysis* (Geneva, 1980).

decade worldwide interruption of smallpox transmission seemed to have been achieved. The success against smallpox encouraged this cadre of organizations – with support from the World Bank Group, other international institutions, and nongovernmental organizations – to establish in 1974 an "Expanded Programme on Immunization" (EPI) aimed at immunizing every child in the world against diphtheria, pertussis, tetanus, measles, poliomyelitis, and tuberculosis by 1990.[66]

By the late 1980s the EPI had achieved substantial success. More than 60 percent of the world's children were by that time receiving immunization against the six target diseases. With success in this initial campaign appearing to be within reach, WHO and its supporting organizations began to look to other serious diseases of the developing world. These included *Haemophilus influenzae* and hepatitis B infection, both diseases against which Merck had already developed effective vaccines.[67]

But Merck and other American vaccine firms had problems in selling vaccines to the EPI. Merck was unable to produce *Recombivax HB* at a cost that would make the new vaccine available in the developing countries. With the new technology, there were opportunities to realize economies of scale over the long term, but in the short run,

---

66 Ibid. J. W. Hopkins, "The Eradication of Smallpox: Organizational Learning and Innovation in International Health Administration," *Journal of Developing Areas* 22 (Apr. 1988): 321–32. World Health Organization, "Immunology: Programme Review, 1963–1969," *World Health Organization Official Records* 182 (1970): 122–34. "Saving Lives by Immunization," *World Health Organization Chronicle* 33 (1979): 128–30. R. H. Henderson, "Vaccine Preventable Diseases of Children: The Problem," in *Protecting the World's Children: Vaccines and Immunization Within Primary Health Care* (New York, 1984), pp. 1–15.

67 B. R. Bloom, "Vaccines for the Third World," *Nature* 342 (Nov. 9, 1989): 115–20. R. H. Henderson, "Global Overview: The Expanded Programme on Immunization," in *Protecting the World's Children: 'Bellagio II' at Cartagena, Colombia, October 1985* (New York, 1986), pp. 13–33. In the same volume see K. S. Warren, "Under the Volcano: The Inevitable New Age of Vaccines," pp. 151-61.

Merck had not yet achieved its economic objective of significantly lowering the price of the HBV vaccine.[68]

If the company placed bids for this vaccine and others at very low prices in the so-called donor market, Merck was attacked in the United States for not offering the same prices in the domestic market. Given the large global demand for vaccines, it was impossible for the company to do with vaccines what it did with *Mectizan*, its treatment for river blindness (onchocerciasis) – that is, give the drug away.[69] For Merck, the U.S. market – and especially the nongovernmental market – provided the firm with the primary opportunities it had to make a return on its investment in vaccines.[70] Even more complex were the problems of stimulating the interest of Merck and other U.S. vaccine producers in research on new vaccines that (like *Mectizan*) had virtually no market outside of the developing countries.[71]

The problems Merck faced in the developing world were similar in some respects to the situations confronting the company in most of the markets of the industrialized countries of Europe and Asia. There too, the primary purchasers were governments, and public con-

---

68 Department of Health and Human Services, "Report on the United States Vaccine Industry" (June 14, 1995), p. 27. With the hepatitis B vaccines, royalties constituted 13–15 percent of sales and were twice the costs of labor and depreciation. Royalties did *not* decline with increased sales.

69 J. L. Sturchio, "The Decision to Donate *Mectizan*: Historical Background." "*Mectizan* (Ivermectin) and the Control of Onchocerciasis: Strengthening the Global Impact" (Rahway, NJ, 1992), Summary Proceedings of the Symposium. J. L. Sturchio to E. English, Mar. 8, 1991. All in MA. E. Eckholm, "River Blindness: Conquering an Ancient Scourge," *New York Times Magazine*, Jan. 8, 1989.

70 A. Robbins and P. Freeman, "Obstacles to Developing Vaccines for the Third World," *Scientific American* (Nov. 1988): 126–33. There were also widespread rumors that the bidding process at UNICEF was corrupt; because U.S. firms could not pay bribes without violating the law, they were effectively eliminated from this part of the donor market.

71 Violaine S. Mitchell, Nalini M. Philipose, and Jay P. Sanford, eds., *The Children's Vaccine Initiative: Achieving the Vision* (Washington, DC, 1993), especially pp. 170–83.

tracts usually resulted in narrow margins – as they did in the United States. The national markets were usually two-tiered: with a large public sector and a smaller private sector in which prices and margins were higher. Only in the United States was the private portion of the market large enough to enable a producer to make profits that would justify continued investment in vaccines over the long run. Only in the United States did Merck not face conditions that favored competing national producers of vaccine products – some of them subsidized by their governments.

These were difficult situations for CEO Vagelos to ponder as he tried to chart the future for Merck's vaccine business. He had considerable discretionary authority: he and the company were operating from positions of unusual strength by the late 1980s. As president of the Merck Sharp & Dohme Research Laboratories (MSDRL) from 1976 to 1984, Vagelos had successfully led the research operations into the new age of targeted biochemical drug discovery.[72] The resulting breakthroughs included *Vasotec* for treating high blood pressure and congestive heart failure; *Primaxin*, a broad-spectrum antibiotic; and *Mevacor*, a cholesterol-lowering agent – the first drug to intervene successfully in the body's cholesterol synthesis pathway. As Merck's CEO since 1985, Vagelos had brought to his new job the same kind of focused, high-energy management that had transformed MSDRL. Innovation across a broad front of corporate activities – line as well as staff; in manufacturing and marketing as well as the laboratories and clinical operations – marked the company's performance in these years. By

---

72 Gambardella, *Science and Innovation*, carefully analyzes this transition. See also H. Grabowski and J. Vernon, "A New Look at the Returns and Risks to Pharmaceutical R&D," *Management Science* 36, no. 7 (1990): 804–21. H. Grabowski and J. Vernon, "Innovation and Structural Change in Pharmaceuticals and Biotechnology," *Industrial and Corporate Change* 3, no. 2 (1994): 435–49, place the transition in a structural, industry-wide context. See also R. Henderson, "The Evolution of Integrative Capability: Innovation in Cardiovascular Drug Discovery," *Industrial and Corporate Change* 3, no. 3 (1994): 607–30. In Henderson's article, her "Alpha" firm is Merck & Co., Inc., and "Dr. A" is Vagelos.

1986, when *Fortune* magazine's annual poll of business leaders picked Merck as its most admired corporation, there was no doubt that an M.D. could be just as good a preparation for corporate leadership in pharmaceuticals as an M.B.A.[73]

Merck had in these years become the global leader in the pharmaceutical industry. Between 1985 and 1987, the firm's total sales had increased from \$3.5 to slightly over \$5 billion. By 1989 they had reached \$6.5 billion – about half of which were made outside the United States. Net income had jumped from \$906 million in 1987 to \$1.5 billion two years later. During this astonishing five-year period of growth, the firm's stockholders realized a total return (stock price increases plus dividends) of 427 percent. *Fortune*'s financial analysts and business executives continued in 1988 and 1989 to rank the business as the nation's "most admired."

Merck's record of growth was all the more impressive because it took place against a general background of American corporate distress. Global competition had since the late 1960s been steadily eating away the advantages U.S. companies had enjoyed during the post-World War II "American Century." Productivity increases – long the primary engine of U.S. growth – had declined sharply in the 1970s, as had expenditures for industrial research. The new era of intense global competition fostered efforts at reconstruction in both the private and public sectors of American society in the 1980s, a decade of wrenching change for many U.S. citizens and for many of their leading business firms.[74]

---

73 Merck & Co., Inc., *Annual Reports*, 1985–90. Sturchio, ed., *Values and Visions*. See pp. 184–5 for figures on sales and share prices. L. Galambos, "The Authority and Responsibility of the Chief Executive Officer: Shifting Patterns in Large U.S. Enterprises in the Twentieth Century," *Industrial and Corporate Change* 4, no. 1 (1995): 187–203.

74 Paul R. Lawrence and Davis Dyer, *Renewing American Industry: Organizing for Efficiency and Innovation* (New York, 1983). Galambos and Pratt, *Rise of the Corporate Commonwealth*, especially pp. 184–255. Angus Maddison, *Phases of Capitalist Development* (New York, 1982), pp. 38–42, 96–125.

By contrast, Merck had during these same years acquired a strong position as a global leader in pharmaceutical innovation, and the success with *Recombivax HB* indicated that the vaccine organization had retained its capacity to innovate after Maurice Hilleman, its primary scientific leader for many years, had retired. During the 1970s and 1980s, Virus and Cell Biology had broadened its capabilities by successfully developing important bacterial vaccines and by moving into recombinant DNA research and development. There were as well promising vaccines in the pipeline.

But if Merck was going to take full advantage of its capabilities in vaccine innovation, the operation was going to need a new champion and perhaps a new position in the firm's organizational hierarchy. Since 1984, Scolnick had been president of the entire Merck Sharp & Dohme Research Laboratories. He was fully occupied directing the thirty or so areas of research in which MSDRL was then working. The labs had a budget of more than $850 million in 1990, and Scolnick had to preside over R & D conducted in several other countries in addition to the large establishments at Rahway, New Jersey, and West Point, Pennsylvania. While he could continue to provide Virus and Cell Biology with scientific leadership, Scolnick could not give the vaccine operations what they most needed at this time. Vaccines needed strategic direction by an executive who had strong links to the many networks – national and international, public and private – that were having an impact on that business. Vaccines needed a single leader, a spokesperson within the upper echelons of Merck, an effective coordinator, a corporate "champion."

CHAPTER 9

VACCINE INNOVATION IN THE NINETIES: NEW STRATEGIES, NEW OPPORTUNITIES, AND PUBLIC CONFRONTATIONS

HE RECOMBINANT DNA technology and the rapidly developing knowledge of gene activity in viral and bacterial pathogens created intriguing opportunities for vaccine innovation in the early 1990s. In its early phase — and it is still in that stage — this particular science/technology cycle resembled in certain regards the bacteriological revolution of the late nineteenth century — the cycle of innovation that yielded the first serum antitoxins and persuaded the H. K. Mulford Company to venture into the new field of biologicals. During the early phase of both cycles, the opportunities for new therapies seemed boundless, giving rise to numerous, small entrepreneurial companies. In both, there were powerful institutional and social barriers to the successful introduction of innovative biological products. In both, the politics of immunization at times overshadowed both the science and the enterprise of vaccines.[1]

---

1 On the early 1990s see R. W. Ellis, "New Technologies for Making Vaccines," and A. R. Hinman and W. A. Orenstein, "Public Health Considerations," both in Plotkin and Mortimer, eds., *Vaccines*, pp. 867–87, and 903–32, respectively. See also *Science* 260 (May 14, 1993): 937–44; and 265 (Sept. 2, 1994): 1371–1404; this latter series of articles starts out with a pessimistic tone (there are "bumps" in the road, researchers are "crawling," and the latest global initiative "has produced little in the way of tangible results"); but then the normal scientific values and rhetoric reassert themselves (there is "recent progress" to report, and new "prospects" to contemplate, and "rapid advances in this field"). See also C. S.

Of course much had also changed since the 1890s, and we have traced many of those transitions in the previous chapters. By the 1990s, the sciences and technologies were far more complex and were fragmented into a much larger number of subdisciplines. Each subdiscipline had its own body of knowledge, channels of communication, leaders, techniques, and values — that is, its own network. The role of the public sector had changed decisively as well. Governmental and intergovernmental agencies were now formidable participants in vaccine distribution, and in the industry's largest markets, national governments were involved in every aspect of vaccine discovery, testing, manufacturing, and marketing.[2]

In the United States in the post-World War II era, a highly productive mixed system had taken shape. This system combined private, public, and professional networks in ways that contributed to rapid advances in the science, technology, and business of vaccine development. For companies that acquired the capabilities — as Merck did — to be aggressive innovators under these conditions, the postwar era was one of expansion and long-term financial success. But this particular system of institutions was unstable. The professions and their supporting institutions became dependent upon increasing levels of government economic support — a situation that was unlikely to continue unchanged forever.[3] The public components in a very large democracy with a heterogeneous population were also unlikely to remain stable over the long run. And the

---

Reiss and B. T. Rouse, "The Current Status of Viral Immunology," *Immunology Today* 14, no. 7 (1993): 333–5; also 15, no. 4 (1994): 155–9. *Lancet* 335 (June 16, 1990): 1436–8; 345 (Apr. 22, 1995): 999. *Pediatric Clinics of North America* 37, no. 3 (1990): 513–30.

2 Department of Health and Human Services, "Report on the United States Vaccine Industry" (June 14, 1995), pp. 4, 14, 17.

3 Our reference here is to the state and federal support for the research universities that provided professional training and sustained basic research. In the medical sciences, the NIH also played a leading role in supporting basic research.

private sector was subject to market forces that virtually guaranteed change.

In the 1970s and 1980s, the vaccine industry was transformed: now only four major firms provided more than 70 percent of the world's supplies. The climax to the most recent wave in the vaccine concentration movement came in 1989. In November, American Cyanamid acquired Praxis Biologicals, creating Lederle Praxis Biologicals, the third-ranking company in the industry.[4] Then, in the following month, Institut Mérieux acquired Connaught BioSciences, making that organization the largest in the world.[5] With sales of $360 million (21 percent), Merck was now a close second, and SmithKline Biologicals was fourth, with approximately 12 percent of world sales.

Three primary factors were driving these structural changes: the intense price competition that characterized the industry; the closely related search for economies of scale and scope in vaccine research, development, manufacturing, and marketing; and the necessity to remain innovative in order to be profitable. The predictions of Merck's 1979 *Vaccine Study* had turned out to be painfully accurate. The unfortunate economic conditions that had characterized the vaccine industry through the 1970s had continued to present problems for most of the producers in the following decade. Patent protection was narrow and competition intense. Government and intergovernment purchases were substantial, forcing the firms remaining in the business to contend with relatively narrow margins in substantial segments of their markets. The total global market was about $1.7 billion by the end of the decade – compared to more than $120 billion for pharmaceuticals, for which profit margins were larger, liability generally perceived as less of

---

4 Lederle/Praxis had total sales of about $250 million, 15 percent of the world market. This firm has since been acquired by American Home Products.

5 Rhone-Poulenc S. A. owned the controlling share of Institut Mérieux's stock. Institut Mérieux, which also owned Pasteur Vaccins, had total global sales of about $400 million (24 percent of the market).

a problem, and patent protection easier to maintain.[6] These conditions prompted Merck's executives once again to rethink the firm's strategy.

1

The company's strategic analysis in 1991 gave only passing consideration to the possibility of leaving the vaccine business. This was a Vagelos-era study that gave overriding consideration to the medical viewpoint that prevention was the best cure. As Merck's internal study group noted, the first element in the Merck statement of corporate purpose was "to provide society with superior products – innovations that improve the quality of life. . . . It is in this context that the Mission of Merck's Vaccine Business must be seen."[7] There was also a political rationale for not seriously considering divestiture. By the 1990s, Merck and the other leading firms were deeply enmeshed in the vaccine networks and had acquired important public and professional obligations. "How would governmental and financial observers view our exit from a high profile scientific field?" the study asked. The report suggested that there might be a "fire storm of criticism" that would spill over onto the firm's other enterprises.

Instead of divestiture, the study focused primarily on how strong Merck's support for vaccines should be and concluded that the company should make a substantial investment in building that part of its business. Actually, it already had. In 1989 Merck had decided to construct two live-virus vaccine laboratories and support operations.

---

6 For a different estimate ($3 billion) of the global market in 1992, see Department of Health and Human Services, "Report on the United States Vaccine Industry" (June 14, 1995), p. 7.

7 As the statement and the group both observed, the company also had to provide its "investors with a superior rate of return" and its employees with "meaningful work." This and all subsequent references to and quotations from the report refer to Merck & Co., Inc., "Vaccine Business . . . Strategic Plan," Jan. 21, 1991. The Vaccine Planning Group that conducted the study included: G. M. Brodhead, C. B. Clarke, G. M. Crooks, R. G. Douglas, D. G. Dunn, A. Y. Elliott, E. A. Fagan, D. L. Litvinas, K. Maher, M. B. Mitchell, T. Poirot, J. L. Ryan, and B. A. Senich.

The following year the company approved an automation project for one of its new vaccines and adopted a capital plan that included a significant new vaccine/biological facility at West Point, Pennsylvania. Momentum was on the side of Virus and Cell Biology, and the 1991 study was consistent with these earlier initiatives.

Support for a significant level of investment was provided by the performance of Merck's workhorse vaccine for measles, mumps, and rubella. Hilleman and his coworkers had improved the original product, replacing Merck's rubella vaccine with the RA 27/3 strain of virus developed by Dr. Stanley Plotkin.[8] The new combination, *M-M-R II*, had since 1979 occupied a central place in the pediatric market – a market that in turn occupied a crucial position in the firm's total vaccine sales. There were no domestic competitors for this product. In 1989, when a dramatic upsurge in measles prompted a medical recommendation for a second dose of vaccine, the company initially found it difficult to keep up with the demand.[9]

---

8 M. R. Hilleman, "Past, Present, and Future of Measles, Mumps, and Rubella Virus Vaccines," *Pediatrics* 90, no. 1 (1992): 149–53. Plotkin's strain of the rubella virus produced less arthropathy in adult women and after 1979 was the only licensed rubella vaccine in this country. S. A. Plotkin, "Rubella Vaccine," in Plotkin and Mortimer, eds., *Vaccines*, pp. 310–11; see also p. 241. R. E. Weibel, A. J. Carlson, Jr., V. M. Villarejos, E. B. Buynak, A. A. McLean, and M. R. Hilleman, "Clinical and Laboratory Studies of Combined Live Measles, Mumps, and Rubella Vaccines Using the RA 27/3 Rubella Virus," *Proceedings of the Society for Experimental Biology and Medicine* 165 (1980): 323–6. See also *Journal of Biological Standardization* 8 (1980): 281–7. "Medical Background: Measles, Mumps, and Rubella," Apr. 1990, MA.

9 American Academy of Pediatrics, Committee on Infectious Diseases, "Measles: Reassessment of the Current Immunization Policy," *Pediatrics* 84, no. 6 (1989): 1110–13. R. R. Wittler, B. C. Veit, S. McIntyre, and M. Schydlower, "Measles Revaccination Response in a School-Age Population," *Pediatrics* 88, no. 5 (1991): 1024–30. See also: *MMWR* 38, no. S-9 (1989): 1–18. *Pediatric Clinics of North America* 37, no. 3 (1990): 603–25, 651–68. *JAMA* 266, no. 8 (1991): 1077–8. *Pediatrics* 89, no. 4 (1992): 589–92. *Bulletin of the World Health Organization* 71, no. 1 (1993): 93–103. Merck & Co., Inc., *Extract* (May/June 1991): 2–8, MA.

M-M-R II and other combination vaccines played a crucial role in the world market and were likely to become even more important in the years ahead. As of 1990, 86 percent of the global market was in the United States, Europe, and Japan; three vaccines (measles-mumps-rubella; diphtheria-pertussis-tetanus; and oral or injectable polio) made up 70 percent of worldwide sales.[10] To extend the market, biological firms and public health organizations would have to promote vaccination in less developed areas where the logistical and economic problems were formidable. In those areas, combination vaccines were a vital means of reducing the social cost and increasing the probability of vaccination. In order to hold its strong position in the U.S. market and gain a larger share of markets in the rest of the world, Merck would have to develop new combination vaccines – especially those for pediatric use.[11]

The study group recommended three significant initiatives. Merck, the group concluded, should organize a separate business unit headed by a "champion" for vaccines. Some years before, the company had reached the same conclusion about its animal health business. The reasoning in both cases was similar.[12] When vaccines were marketed through the normal channels – that is, MSD in the United States and Merck Sharp & Dohme International (MSDI) overseas – they competed for time and attention with pharmaceuticals. Since the pharmaceutical business was much larger, vaccines tended to get squeezed out. Within the firm and without, vaccines needed an "advocate," a leader who could deal effectively with the complex political and economic environment for this business. Merck needed an "identifiable" spokesperson

---

10 All of these figures are for sales in dollars; the percentages would of course be very different if we were using units or doses of vaccines distributed.

11 See also Department of Health and Human Services, "Report on the United States Vaccine Industry" (June 14, 1995), especially p. 2.

12 James Gillin, Oral History, July 18, 1990, MA.

who could tend the relevant vaccine networks. It also needed a strong executive who would ensure that the firm's research, manufacturing, and marketing efforts for vaccines were coordinated.

The vaccine unit should, the study group said, implement a new strategy emphasizing alliances and licensing – an external growth strategy – as a means of broadening Merck's product line. Since the company did not have a diphtheria-tetanus-pertussis vaccine for combination purposes, Merck should look to one of its competitors for that important pediatric vaccine. Merck was already taking this approach to growth in its pharmaceutical business.[13] Alliances with AB Astra, Johnson & Johnson, and Du Pont enabled Merck to extend its research and marketing capabilities without paying premium prices to acquire other businesses.[14] In vaccines, the ideal partner appeared to be Mérieux/Connaught, but there were other combinations that might also be successful.

To make the new structure and strategy successful, the study group said, Merck should increase its investments in vaccines. Research and development needed additional support to maintain a "broad-based capability for developing and registering vaccine candidates." The right kind of strategic alliance might help with production, as well as marketing and governmental relations overseas. If Merck was willing to build its vaccine capabilities in this way, the study said, the financial returns

---

13 During the administrations of Ronald Reagan and George Bush, the U.S. government had virtually abandoned the structural side of the federal antitrust policy. This made it possible for large firms in concentrated industries to implement joint ventures of the sort Merck had launched with Johnson & Johnson and Du Pont. Merck & Co., Inc., *1989 Annual Report*, pp. 4, 22; *1990 Annual Report*, pp. 6, 41–3.

14 F. H. Spiegel, Jr., "Johnson & Johnson ∘ Merck Consumer Pharmaceuticals Co." Apr. 19, 1990, MA. W. Koberstein, "Joseph Mollica," *Pharmaceutical Executive* (May 1991): 25–32. *Wall Street Journal*, July 26, 1990. Merck & Co., Inc., *1990 Annual Report*, pp. 41–5. In vaccines, Merck brought to the combinations its licensed products plus its substantial development capabilities.

would enable the company "to remain a viable participant in this market over the long term."

2

The new vaccine study gave Roy Vagelos and the Merck Board of Directors a solid rationale for organizing the Merck Vaccine Division, and the study group also provided the division's "champion." R. Gordon Douglas, Jr., M.D. – an authority on infectious diseases – had served from 1982 through 1989 as chairman of the Department of Medicine at Cornell University's Medical College.[15] In 1990 Douglas had joined Merck as a senior vice president for medical and scientific affairs in the international division and in that capacity became a member of the vaccine study group. In March 1991, Vagelos appointed him president of the new division.

Aside from making some key appointments, Gordon Douglas's first priority was to establish the strategic alliances that were central to the division's future. Following the blueprint of the 1991 strategic plan, he first targeted Connaught Laboratories, Inc., a subsidiary of Pasteur Mérieux Serums & Vaccins. The two organizations complemented each other well. Merck could provide *PedvaxHIB* (against Haemophilus influenzae Type b) and *Recombivax HB* (against hepatitis B), neither of which Connaught had access to in the U.S. market. Connaught's blue chips were DTP and a polio vaccine, both of which were important for any

---

15 A graduate of the Cornell University Medical College in 1959, Douglas interned at New York Hospital and served his residency at that institution and at the Johns Hopkins Hospital in Baltimore, Maryland. He was a clinical investigator at the National Institutes of Health, NIAID, from 1963 to 1966. He subsequently was a faculty member at the Baylor College of Medicine (1966–70) and the University of Rochester School of Medicine (1970–82). Douglas is coeditor of and contributor to one of the leading reference works in his field: Mandell, Douglas, and Bennett, eds., *Principles and Practice of Infectious Diseases*. He had published extensively on various aspects of bacteriological and viral infections in humans, including in particular those caused by influenza viruses. Like Hilleman, Douglas had for years been active in many of the national and international organizations in the virology, bacteriology, and immunology networks.

combination pediatric product. The two firms quickly agreed to collaborate in the research, development, manufacturing, and marketing of pediatric combination vaccines.[16]

Other agreements along the same lines followed in the next few years, gradually extending the division's reach. In 1992, the company's Australian subsidiary joined with Commonwealth Serum Laboratories (CSL) in marketing pediatric combination vaccines in Australia, New Zealand, and the Pacific Rim.[17] Looking to Asian markets that appeared to have substantial growth potential, the division next completed a development and marketing agreement with Japan's Chemo-Sero-Therapeutic Research Institute (Kaketsuken).[18] In Europe, Merck built on the foundation provided by the collaboration with Connaught. In 1993, Connaught's parent firm, Mérieux, agreed to establish a joint venture (Pasteur Mérieux MSD) to promote the existing and future vaccines of Merck and Mérieux in Europe and to develop additional combination products.[19] As a result, the division had at a reasonable price significantly extended its R & D, manufacturing, and marketing capabilities, and also opened new avenues for future growth.[20]

---

16 Merck & Co., Inc., *1992 Annual Report*, p. 17.

17 Ibid. Merck & Co., Inc., *The Daily*, Nov. 10, 1992, MA. Commonwealth, which was in the course of privatization, changed its name to CSL. *Scrip*, Oct. 27, 1992.

18 Merck & Co., Inc., *1994 Annual Report*, p. 23. In 1993, the division also signed an agreement with Korea Green Cross Corporation, South Korea's leading vaccine company. Korea Green Cross sold Merck's *Pneumovax 23* and *PedvaxHIB*.

19 *La Tribune*, July 15, 1993. Merck & Co., Inc., *1993 Annual Report*, p. 22. The European Commission approved this joint venture in October 1994; the new organization, with headquarters in Lyon, France, now does business in nineteen European countries. *Business Wire*, Oct. 6, 1994. *AP-Dow Jones News*, July 6, 1993. *Scrip*, July 15, 1993. Merck & Co., Inc., *1994 Annual Report*, p. 23.

20 For example, the Australian agreement with CSL Limited was originally designed to cover pediatric vaccines. By 1994, however, the two companies had also completed another agreement to codevelop a vaccine to prevent sexually

While strengthening its position in the developed world, the vaccine division found it difficult to improve in any marked way its contribution to the donor market. Merck was producing without subsidies. While the firm bid on selected contracts at prices lower than those in the United States, there was pressure from Congress to set one price for the overseas markets and for the public health markets at home.[21] Moreover, in 1990, total donor sales by all firms – sales to UNICEF, to PAHO, and to AID – constituted only 4 percent of the global market (in dollars). The World Summit for Children in that year launched a Children's Vaccine Initiative (CVI) to increase immunization levels with the support of the United Nations, the World Bank Group, the World Health Organization, and the Rockefeller Foundation. Although Merck participated in the initiative's working groups, the company could not overcome the basic political and economic barriers that limited U.S. private-sector contributions to this campaign.[22]

More successful were Merck's efforts to assist the Romanian and Chinese governments in meeting their vaccine needs. Following the collapse of East European communism, many of the nations in that region had serious public health problems.[23] In 1992, Merck cooper-

---

transmitted diseases that were linked to cervical cancer. Merck & Co., Inc., *1994 Annual Report*, p. 23.

21 Department of Health and Human Services, "Report on the United States Vaccine Industry" (June 14, 1995), pp. 4, 10.

22 Mitchell, Philipose, and Sanford, eds., *Children's Vaccine Initiative*, especially pp. 2–18, 31–3, 49–50, 128–45. A. R. Pebley, "Goals of the World Summit for Children and Their Implications for Health Policy in the 1990s," in James N. Gribble and Samuel H. Preston, eds., *The Epidemiological Transition: Policy and Planning Implications for Developing Countries* (Washington, DC, 1993), pp. 170–96.

23 On some of the Russian problems see *Science* 261 (July 23, 1993): 415. *TASS*, July 27, 1993. *Reuters, Ltd.*, Aug. 4, 1993. *New York Times*, Aug. 22, 1993. *Financial Times*, Aug. 19, 1993.

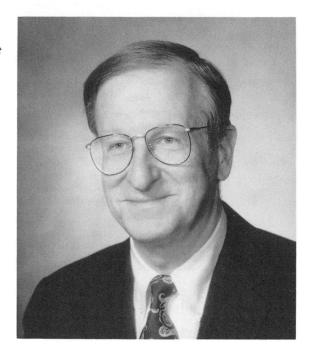

R. Gordon Douglas, Jr., M.D., President of Merck Vaccines.

ated with the international health organization Project HOPE in vaccinating Romanian children against hepatitis B and in conducting educational conferences to encourage immunization. In this case, the company donated more than 125,000 doses of *Recombivax HB*.[24]

Merck assisted the People's Republic of China in building facilities to make a genetically engineered hepatitis B vaccine on terms that were significantly more generous than a normal commercial transaction. The negotiations over this form of technology transfer were prolonged. But hepatitis B infection and the related problems of liver cancer were China's greatest health problems, and both sides persisted through this extended exercise in commercial diplomacy. The final result, in 1993, was one of the most up-to-date vaccine facilities in the world. Merck

---

24 C. Paquet, V. T. Babes, J. Drucker, B. Senemaud, and A. Dobrescu, "Viral Hepatitis in Bucharest," *Bulletin of the World Health Organization* 71, no. 6 (1993): 781–6. Merck & Co., Inc., *1991 Contributions Report*, pp. 10–11; Press releases, Mar. 16 and 18, 1992; and enclosure in P. V. Maehara to L. Schwartz, June 16, 1992; all in MA.

engineers trained their Chinese counterparts at the units in the United States, then shipped the facilities to China to be reassembled.[25]

4

At home during the 1990s, Merck's new vaccine division suddenly became the focal point of an angry, frustrating political debate. Merck and its leadership, including Gordon Douglas, president of the division, found themselves caught in a political struggle that was in many ways more intense than the Kefauver Hearings of the late 1950s and early 1960s. The company had tried for some years to anticipate these problems, to shape a political economy that was not hostile to private enterprise in general and to pharmaceutical companies in particular. The entire healthcare industry was experiencing a major transformation during the 1980s and early 1990s, and changes of this magnitude always attract political attention in the United States. This was especially true in this instance because substantial government programs − Medicare and Medicaid, for example − were directly involved in the changes taking place. The fact that significant numbers of Americans were not protected by health insurance during this era of transition made it all the more likely that healthcare reform would become one of the primary political issues of the 1990s.[26]

It was in that volatile context that CEO Vagelos arranged to let Democratic candidate Bill Clinton speak at Merck's Rahway, New Jersey, headquarters during the 1992 presidential campaign. While Clinton's September talk called for price controls on prescription drugs, Merck had anticipated that issue as early as 1990 by pledging to limit its overall price increases to the rate of inflation. Besides, Clinton seemed to want fewer, not more, government efforts "to micromanage health care."[27] After Clinton's November election victory, Vagelos and

---

25 Merck, press release, June 9, 1994, and accompanying materials, MA.

26 See, for instance, *Pediatrics* 89, no. 5 (1992): 983–98; 89, no. 6 (1992): 1019–26.

27 *New York Times*, Sept. 25, 1992.

his political advisers within the company knew that the incoming administration would make healthcare reform a major goal in its program, but they had good reason to believe that the reform effort would not impinge in any dramatic way on the pharmaceutical industry or Merck & Co., Inc.

They were wrong. Once the Clinton Administration was up and running, the dynamics of liberal ideology, of interest-group action, and of bureaucratic politics combined to create an environment extremely hostile to the pharmaceutical industry and especially to its largest firms. The Administration first singled out vaccine producers for special attention, apparently hoping to use vaccine reform as the entering wedge for changes in the general healthcare system.[28] In the short term, this appeared to be an astute political decision. There were only four major producers in the world and those in the United States were both branches of large, successful firms. Merck had experienced substantial growth in its pharmaceutical operations in recent years. Its vaccine business had continued to be profitable too, although as we have seen in the previous chapters, the profit margins had always been narrow relative to pharmaceuticals.

Accuracy notwithstanding, however, the politics of vaccines favored the Administration, which shrewdly emphasized the important shots that were not being given to children. The low immunization rates in the United States, the Administration said, were a product of high prices charged by powerful corporations. "Our prices are shocking," Clinton said.[29] This style of political rhetoric appealed to several traditional Democratic constituencies, as it had during the Progressive Era and the New Deal of the 1930s.[30]

---

28 *Associated Press*, Feb. 1, 1993. *New York Post*, Feb. 2, 1993. *Washington Post*, Feb. 2, 1993.

29 *New York Times*, Feb. 13, 1993. *Baltimore Sun* Feb. 13, 1993. *Miami Herald*, Feb. 13, 1993. *Wall Street Journal*, Feb. 23 and 24, 1993.

30 The measles epidemic of 1989–90 also helped make this issue politically effective. *JAMA* 266, no. 11 (1991): 1547–52.

The Clinton assault left Gordon Douglas and the vaccine division scrambling to defend their enterprise, one in which Merck had just recently reaffirmed its commitment and decided to make major investments. Douglas and his colleagues were not without allies or intellectual ammunition. It was, after all, high liability and tighter profit margins – not price gouging – that had driven most of the other pharmaceutical firms out of vaccines entirely. High profits normally have the opposite effect in a market economy. Moreover, public health officials and academicians knew that America's low immunization levels were not a result of high prices. Parents failed to have their children properly vaccinated even when the shots were free, as they were for a significant part of the population. To a considerable extent the nation's clinics, HMOs, and private-practice physicians were responsible for this problem and for the many "missed opportunities" to vaccinate children.[31]

Educational programs and public health outreach plans at the state and local levels were needed, as Douglas and public health professionals tried to make clear during the ensuing political debate. The vaccine division had already launched several initiatives, including support for local projects to improve immunization rates and a program to reduce acquisition costs of vaccines for children covered by Medicaid.[32] As the political controversy intensified, Douglas applauded the Administration's plan to spend more on vaccines, but he warned that in states with large public programs the "immunization rates are no higher than states without such programs."[33]

---

31 See, for instance, Johns Hopkins University and the University of Maryland, *The Baltimore Immunization Study: Immunization Coverage and Causes of Under-Immunization Among Inner-City Children in Baltimore* ([Baltimore], 1993). *New England Journal of Medicine* 327, no. 25 (1992): 1794–1800. *Associated Press*, Feb. 20, 1993. *Philadelphia Inquirer*, Feb. 20, 1993. *Health Line*, Feb. 8, 1993. *Washington Post*, Feb. 10, 1993. *Pediatrics* 91, no. 1 (1993): 1–7.

32 Merck & Co., Inc., *1992 Annual Report*, p. 17.

33 *New York Times*, Feb. 13, 1993. See also *New York Times*, Feb. 14, 1993; and

During this brief struggle, the Clinton Administration's long-term goal appears to have been a national vaccine agency in which political authority would largely, if not entirely, supplant market forces. The 1985 study by the Institute of Medicine and the 1993 study stemming from the Children's Summit had advanced proposals along these lines.[34] Neither study gave much attention to the advantages over the long term of a mixed system that combined public, nonprofit professional, and profit-seeking institutions in a manner that achieved specialization of function and employed market constraints to ensure efficiency. Neither study recognized that public institutions, like those in the private sector, experience cycles of innovation of the sort we have observed in the previous chapters.[35] Nor did they acknowledge that adequate returns to innovation would accelerate new vaccine development in the private sector.[36] The Clinton Administration appears to have taken a similar tack in developing its new plan for U.S. vaccine distribution.

Most revealing in this regard was the Administration effort to

---

Pediatrics 91, no. 2 (1993): 308–14 and 315–20; 91, no. 3 (1993): 605–11. There were in some cases differences, and the question was, then, whether those differences were significant.

34 See also *JAMA* 270, no. 15 (1993): 1782, 1784.

35 See Chapters 2, 5, and 8, above. See also D. Milobsky and L. Galambos, "The McNamara Bank and Its Legacy, 1968–1987" (forthcoming, *Business and Economic History* 24, no. 2 [1995]) for a perspective on long cycles of innovation at that public institution. The history of the Tennessee Valley Authority is also instructive in this regard.

36 This issue came up in the great vaccine debate of 1993. See, for instance, *New York Times*, Apr. 2, 1993. See also *Health Line*, July 2, 1993. An exception to this generalization is provided by B. R. Bloom, "The United States Needs a National Vaccine Authority," *Science* 265 (Sept. 2, 1994): 1378–80. Bloom noted that "problems with liability and profitability" had sharply reduced the number of private firms in the industry. "Recognizing that monopolies inevitably place the public interest at risk, I believe that interest is best served by multiple manufacturers and competition, not by monopsonistic or universal government purchase, which will limit development of new and improved vaccines."

purchase the entire supply of pediatric vaccines in the United States.[37] Monopsony would supplant oligopsony, and the assumption was that greater efficiency and equity would be achieved, to the advantage of the American public.[38]

Merck and its professional, commercial, and political allies were able to put a dent in this part of the Administration's program.[39] At this point in the controversy, the firm's well tended relationships with the public health, scientific, and medical networks came into play. The United States did not end up with central, federal direction — something along the lines of the Institute of Medicine's proposed national vaccine commission or agency — for the industry.[40] Professional critiques helped to shoot holes in this part of the Administration's proposal.[41]

But it was impossible to stop the entire drive for a new program. The President's knowledge of pediatrics may have been flawed, but not

37 *New York Times*, Apr. 1, 1993. *Washington Post*, Apr. 1, 1993. The idea had been floated in February of that year. *Washington Times*, Feb. 2, 1993.

38 *New York Times*, Feb. 1, 1993. See the editorial in support of the program in *New York Times*, Feb. 2, 1993.

39 *Science* 259 (Mar. 12, 1993): 1529. *Washington Post*, Apr. 2, 1993.

40 There was a strong ideological current running in that direction. See, for instance, Institute of Medicine, *Vaccine Supply and Innovation*. Mitchell, Philipose, and Sanford, eds., *Children's Vaccine Initiative*. *Washington Post*, May 6, 1993. *Los Angeles Times*, May 5, 1993. *Philadelphia Inquirer*, May 6, 1993.

41 *Pediatrics* 91, no. 1 (1993): 160. G. L. Freed and S. L. Katz, "The Comprehensive Childhood Immunization Act of 1993," *New England Journal of Medicine* 329, no. 26 (1993): 1957–60. *Modern Healthcare*, May 17, 1993. *JAMA* 269, no. 16 (1993): 2062–3. *Pediatric News*, Sept. 1993. *New York Times*, May 5, 1993. See the editorial response in *New York Times*, May 6, 1993. See also *New York Times*, May 16 and Aug. 11, 1993. For an attempt to revive the agency concept see *Science* 261 (July 9, 1993): 156. One of the opponents of this part of the plan was former Surgeon General C. Everett Koop. See also *PR Newswire*, Apr. 7, 1993; *Washington Post*, May 3, 1993; *Boston Globe*, Apr. 27, 1993; *Atlanta Constitution*, July 13, 1993. There was also Republican opposition; see *U.S. Newswire*, May 4, 1993.

his sense of politics. "We cannot have profits at the expense of our children," he said.[42] Neither Merck nor the other vaccine manufacturers could provide an equally appealing sound bite for the evening news. When Gordon Douglas and representatives of the other leading firms in the industry met with the Secretary of Health and Human Services Donna E. Shalala, they defended their price policies. Eighty percent of the price increases for pediatric immunization, Douglas said, were a result of new federal excise taxes and the addition of two new vaccines.[43]

But the steamroller kept moving.[44] Roy Vagelos identified the "real problem" as the existing government programs: "They lack the infrastructure, organizational skills and people needed to get already purchased vaccines to needy children."[45] But Washington was not listening, and the steamroller moved on. Congress passed a scaled-down version of the original Clinton proposal, one that ostensibly provided vaccines only for children who are American Indians, are uninsured, are using community health centers, or are covered by Medicaid.[46] The entitlement was set at $585 million.

While the initial response to the new law was favorable,[47] the

---

42 *New York Times*, Feb. 13 and 25, 1993.

43 *New York Times*, Mar. 2, 1993. These contentions sparked a lively public debate. See, for instance, *New York Times*, Mar. 3 and 15, 1993; *Associated Press*, Mar. 2, 1993; *Science* 259 (Mar. 12, 1993): 1528–9.

44 *New York Times*, Apr. 13, 1993.

45 *New York Times*, Apr. 20, 1993. See also *New York Times*, Apr. 22 and May 2, 1993. *Business Wire*, Apr. 21, 1993. *Dow Jones News Service*, Apr. 21, 1993.

46 *Dow Jones News Service*, May 19, 1993. *SCRIP*, Aug. 17, 1993. *Health Line*, Aug. 24, 1993. George Washington University, *State Health Notes* 14, no. 163 (1993). *New York Times*, June 23 and Aug. 16, 1993. We say "ostensibly" because there were no controls on access. See Vagelos's parting shot at the measure in *New York Times*, Aug. 28, 1993.

47 See the optimistic reports in *JAMA* 272, no. 15 (1994): 1156–7; 272, no. 17 (1994): 1316–17; *Pediatrics* 94, no. 4 (1994): 545–7.

Administration's public initiative soon attracted some strong criticism.[48] Some of the early critiques were prompted by the Administration's effort to return to its original plan by simply buying up 60 to 65 percent of the domestic supply of pediatric vaccines. Apparently the initial plan was to store these delicate biologicals in a government warehouse in Burlington, New Jersey, from which they could be distributed throughout the nation. Even Senator Dale Bumpers (Democrat of Arkansas), a strong proponent of immunization, was critical: "I sense an impending train wreck," he said. "It's very dangerous to store so much of our nation's vaccine supply in one facility."[49] Despite assurances by the Secretary of Health and Human Services that "our piece of this program is in good shape," the General Accounting Office (GAO) concluded in the summer of 1994 that the entire Vaccines for Children (VFC) program was in deep trouble. The Administration's program, the GAO said, would probably not achieve its major objective, increasing immunization levels.[50] The

---

48 See, for example, *New York Times*, Apr. 24 and May 15, 1995. *Associated Press*, Apr. 3, 1995. For a more gentle critique see *Pediatrics* 93, no. 3 (1994): 373–8; 94, no. 1 (1994): 53–8; 94, no. 3 (1994): 376–80. *JAMA* 269, no. 12 (1993): 1480–1; 272, no. 14 (1994): 1111–15.

49 *New York Times*, May 30, 1994. See also the comment by Dr. Michael T. Osterhold, the state epidemiologist in Minnesota: "It's turning into a nightmare for public health officials and private doctors and nurses. We've taken an already complicated system and made it more complicated."

50 U.S. General Accounting Office, "Vaccines for Children: Critical Issues in Design and Implementation" (July 18, 1994), especially pp. 2–4. As the report noted, the Centers for Disease Control were using the General Services Administration for distribution purposes. "GSA has no experience with storing, packaging, and delivering vaccines, and although they have contracted with Federal Express for the *delivery* of vaccines, officials told us they had neither plans nor formal arrangements to test shipping containers and their performance during delivery" (p. 3). See also *New York Times*, July 17, 1994; and *JAMA* 272, no. 8 (1994): 576–7.

Administration dropped the New Jersey warehouse plan shortly after this initial report.[51]

The final GAO report followed, however, and concluded that "the cost to parents of vaccines has not been a major barrier to children's timely immunization."[52] The GAO's "scathing audit" undercut the rationale for VFC, blunted the Administration's effort to achieve general healthcare reform, and provided support for those who were trying to defend a mixed system with a strong private component as a source of vaccine innovations.[53]

---

51 *New York Times*, Aug. 23, 1995. Senator Bumpers commented: "A fairly simple law, designed to benefit a relatively small group of uninsured children, was transformed into a bureaucratic nightmare that put the safety and availability of a third of our nation's vaccine supply at risk." See the editorial in *New York Times*, Aug. 24, 1994.

52 U.S. General Accounting Office, "Vaccines for Children: Reexamination of Program Goals and Implementation Needed to Ensure Vaccination" (June 15, 1995), p. 1. The GAO found that "CDC-sponsored studies clearly demonstrate that, since underimmunized children generally had access to free vaccine before VFC began, cost is less important than missed opportunities for vaccination during their regular contacts with their health care providers" (p. 6).

53 *New York Times*, June 25, 1995. See also the Administration's defense in *New York Times*, June 26, 1995, and the negative evaluation in Robert M. Goldberg, *The Vaccines for Children Program: A Critique* (Washington, DC, 1995). Our evaluation is consistent with Department of Health and Human Services, "Report on the United States Vaccine Industry" (June 14, 1995). On the failure of general healthcare reform see the "Roundtable on the Defeat of Reform," *Journal of Health Politics, Policy and Law* 20, no. 2 (1995): 391–494.

The authors of this book do not completely agree about the relative roles of private and public-sector contributions to innovation. In the spirit of Joseph A. Schumpeter, Sewell (a British citizen) has substantial faith in the ability of public institutions to provide the medical innovations we need. Galambos (a U.S. citizen) has substantial faith in markets as the best means of ensuring that our institutions will remain innovative over the long term. The authors do agree that a mixed system will probably always be optimal, especially in the United States.

5

Over the long term, of course, Merck and the industry's best defense against similar threats to the mixed system was the ability to sustain innovation in vaccine development and delivery. With that objective in mind, Merck substantially enhanced its vaccine development capabilities, adding new personnel and constructing a new biotechnology manufacturing complex at West Point, Pennsylvania. One of the products of this increased investment on the development side of R & D was a new vaccine for chicken pox.

Because the three major pediatric vaccines had been so successful, chicken pox had become the most common of the childhood diseases by the 1990s.[54] Each year there were three to four million cases in the United States. While complications were less likely than with other childhood diseases, they could include encephalitis or varicella pneumonia.[55] Chicken pox was much more severe in immunosuppressed individuals, and part of the enthusiasm for a vaccine stemmed from the needs of this group of patients.[56] There were, however, some complicating aspects in dealing with this virus. *Herpesvirus varicellae* caused both chicken pox and herpes zoster, an inflammation of the sensory nerves seen largely among adults. Herpes zoster (commonly called shingles) was associated with previous varicella infections and an alteration in the immunologic system that resulted in the activation of the latent virus.[57] Zoster immune globulin had been used successfully to provide passive immunization against chicken pox, but physicians could not

54 The three major pediatric vaccines were those for measles, mumps, and rubella; for diphtheria, tetanus, and pertussis; and for polio.

55 S. Krugman, "Varicella and Herpes Virus Infections," in William L. Bradford, ed., *Symposium on Infectious Diseases* (Philadelphia, 1960), pp. 881–902.

56 The mortality rate in immunosuppressed children was estimated to be approximately 7 percent. C. J. White and S. A. Plotkin, "Varicella Vaccine," MA.

57 E. Gold, "Serologic and Virus-Isolation Studies of Patients with Varicella or Herpes-Zoster Infection," *New England Journal of Medicine* 274, no. 4 (1966): 181–5.

*Project Hope: Merck
donated vaccine being
used in Roumania.*

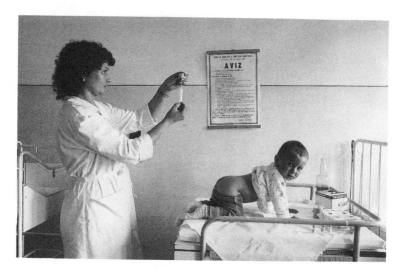

prevent the disease nor could they ensure that herpes zoster would not
follow the attack many years later.

In the 1970s, researchers had turned their attention to vaccines.[58] Dr. M. Takahashi in Japan isolated the Oka strain of virus and
attenuated it successfully in tissue cultures.[59] Clinical tests indicated
that his vaccine was effective and produced minimal side effects.[60] In
the meantime, Hilleman and his associates had isolated and attenuated
a different strain of varicella (KMcC) but had not achieved the results

58 P. A. Brunell, A. Ross, L. H. Miller, and B. Kuo, "Prevention of Varicella by
Zoster Immune Globulin," *New England Journal of Medicine* 280, no. 22 (1969):
1191–4; see also pp. 1237–8. Passive immunization was used with
immunodeficient children and adults.

59 *Lancet* (Nov. 30, 1974): 1288, 1300–1. See also *Lancet* (May 1, 1976): 965;
and *Pediatrics* 59, no. 1 (1977): 1–2, 3–7, 8–12.

60 See *Pediatrics* 59, no. 1 (1977): 1–2, 3–7, 8–12; 60, no. 6 (1977): 805–9,
810–14; 61, no. 4 (1978): 550–5. See also *Pediatrics* 65, no. 2 (1980): 346–50.

they sought in the early clinical trials.[61] In 1981, Merck licensed the Oka strain from Japan and after further attenuating the virus, prepared a vaccine and launched clinical trials in cooperation with the Department of Pediatrics at the University of Pennsylvania. In the years that followed, the clinical teams gave more than 5,000 children the Oka/Merck vaccine, which proved to be "generally well tolerated, immunogenic, and efficacious."[62]

From the very first, however, the chicken pox vaccine prompted controversy. Most new vaccines have encountered resistance, sometimes from physicians, frequently from public authorities, and almost always from the general population. Merck's pneumonia vaccine, *Pneumovax 23*, had failed to have the impact that the firm and many public health officials had anticipated because of resistance on all three levels.[63] With

---

61 B. J. Neff, R. E. Weibel, V. M. Villarejos, E. B. Buynak, A. A. McLean, D. H. Morton, B. S. Wolanski, and M. R. Hilleman, "Clinical and Laboratory Studies of KMcC Strain Live Attenuated Varicella Virus," *Proceedings of the Society for Experimental Biology and Medicine* 166 (1981): 339–47. See also *Pediatrics* 71, no. 3 (1983): 307–12; 75, no. 4 (1985): 667-71; Merck & Co., Inc., *The Daily*, Mar. 17, 1995.

62 C. J. White and S. A. Plotkin, "Varicella Vaccine," MA. C. J. White, B. J. Kuter, C. S. Hildebrand, K. L. Isganitis, H. Matthews, W. J. Miller, P. J. Provost, R. W. Ellis, R. J. Gerety, and G. B. Calandra, "Varicella Vaccine (*Varivax*) in Healthy Children and Adolescents: Results from 1987–1989 Clinical Trials," *Pediatrics* 87, no. 5 (1991): 604–10. R. E. Weibel, B. J. Neff, B. J. Kuter, H. A. Guess, C. A. Rothenberger, A. J. Fitzgerald, K. A. Connor, A. A. McLean, M. R. Hilleman, E. B. Buynak, and E. M. Scolnick, "Live Attenuated Varicella Virus Vaccine: Efficacy Trial in Healthy Children," *New England Journal of Medicine* 310, no. 22 (1984): 1409–15; and R. E. Weibel, B. J. Kuter, B. J. Neff, C. A. Rothenberger, A. J. Fitzgerald, K. A. Connor, D. Morton, A. A. McLean, and E. M. Scolnick, "Live Oka/Merck Varicella Vaccine in Healthy Children," *JAMA* 254, no. 17 (1985): 2435–9. See also *JAMA* 325, no. 22 (1991): 1545–50; 252, no. 3 (1984): 355–62; *Pediatrics* 81, no. 4 (1988): 512–18; 82, no. 5 (1988): 810–11; 88, no. 3 (1991): 604–7.

63 This was the conclusion of Robert Austrian's 1991 study. E. D. Shapiro, A. T. Berg, R. Austrian, D. Schroeder, V. Parcells, A. Margolis, R. K. Adair, and J. D. Clemens, "The Protective Efficacy of Polyvalent Pneumococcal Polysaccharide

---

varicella, however, the opposition in the 1980s was unusually intense and lasting.

Two major issues were at stake. One was the seriousness of chicken pox, a disease that did not strike fear in the general population or arouse deep concern on the part of healthcare professionals. There was concern that vaccine-induced immunity would eventually wane, resulting in more chicken pox among adolescents and adults. The disease was more serious later in life.[64] The other substantial issue involved the relationship between chicken pox and herpes zoster. Would vaccination of children leave them more vulnerable to painful attacks of herpes zoster when they were adults? Some of the answers to these questions emerged from the research efforts that gradually produced a better understanding of the relationship between chicken pox and zoster.[65] As this process continued, leaders in the scientific and medical networks slowly moved

Vaccine," *New England Journal of Medicine* 325, no. 21 (1991): 1453–60. See also *JAMA* 270, no. 15 (1993): 1826–31. As Pierce Gardner and William Schaffner pointed out in 1993, "The immunization of adults does not receive the same priority as the immunization of children, although deaths from vaccine-preventable diseases occur predominantly in adults." "Immunization of Adults," *New England Journal of Medicine* 328, no. 17 (1993): 1252–8.

64 For a sample of the exchanges see *JAMA* 238, no. 16 (1977): 1731–3; 239, no. 11 (1978): 1034–5. *Pediatrics* 59, no. 1 (1977): 1–2; 59, no. 6 (1977): 953–4; 60, no. 6 (1977): 930–1; 62, no. 5 (1978): 858. For an initial attempt to develop reliable information on which to base decisions see *Pediatrics* 68, no. 1 (1981): 14–17.

65 See, for instance, *JAMA* 247, no. 17 (1982): 2340–1. *Pediatric Infectious Disease Journal* 1, no. 3 (1982): 164–7; 3, no. 6 (1984): 500–9. *Pediatrics* 75, no. 5 (1985): 989–90; 77, no. 1 (1986): 53–6. *New England Journal of Medicine* 309, no. 23 (1983): 1434–40; 318, no. 9 (1988): 543–8, 573–5; 323, no. 10 (1990): 627–31; 325, no. 22 (1991): 1545–50, and the editorial comment on pp. 1577–9. The follow-up clinical studies were also favorable. *Pediatrics* 72, no. 3 (1983): 291–4; 78, no. 4 (1986): 705–7; the supplement to 78 (1986), was devoted to the varicella vaccine; see, especially, pp. 742–7, on a successful clinical study using a combination of *M-M-R II* and the varicella vaccine; 89, no. 1 (1992): 147–9. *JAMA* 250, no. 16 (1983): 2095–6.

toward acceptance and then enthusiastic support for routine immunization.[66] But the vaccine division still had to struggle with public and professional resistance.

Meanwhile, Virus and Cell Biology and the manufacturing division were confronting problems with production. The varicella vaccine is extremely sensitive to temperature inactivation. The process was, the company noted, "hard to measure, harder to test, and extremely hard to mass produce." In order to achieve the control and timing needed for the incubation, freezing, and sterilizing stages, the company used a new robotic technology with computer controls. In handling a single lot of vaccine, the robots carried out more than 22,400 aseptic manipulations in a process extending over thirty-seven days.[67] This was a difficult production technique to set up and a novel challenge for the regulators who had to approve the process.

On March 17, 1995, the Food and Drug Administration finally licensed *Varivax*. The Committee on Infectious Diseases recommended the new vaccine "for universal use in early childhood and immunization in susceptible older children."[68] For more than a quarter of a century, Merck had continued to support research and development on *Varivax*. Four CEOs – Gadsden, Horan, Vagelos, and now

---

66 See, for example, *New England Journal of Medicine* 325, no. 22 (1991): 1577–8; and 320, no. 14 (1989): 892–7. *Pediatrics* 84, no. 6 (1989): 1097–9; 86, no. 3 (1990): 494; 86, no. 6 (1990): 867–73; 90, no. 1 (1992): 144–8. *JAMA* 268, no. 7 (1992): 851–2. See also *Pediatric Infectious Disease Journal* 6, no. 1 (1987): 33–5; *JAMA* 271, no. 5 (1994): 375–81; and *Pediatrics* 95, no. 5 (1995): 632–8, for studies of the economic impact of chicken pox. Additional studies appeared in *Pediatrics* 79, no. 6 (1987): 922–7; 80, no. 4 (1987): 465–72; 80, no. 6 (1987): 933–6; 84, no. 3 (1989): 418–21; 85, no. 3 (1990): 338–44; 87, no. 2 (1991): 166–70; 90, no. 2 (1992): 216–20; 91, no. 1 (1993): 17–22; 92, no. 6 (1993): 833–7; 94, no. 4 (1994): 524–6. *Lancet* (Sept. 12, 1992): 639–40, was still undecided as to "how to manage primary infection with this 'not-so-benign virus.'" See also *JAMA* 271, no. 22 (1994): 1744–5.

67 Merck & Co., Inc., *The Daily*, Mar. 17, 1995, MA.

68 *Pediatrics* 95, no. 5 (1995): 791–6.

Ray Gilmartin[69] – had directed the firm through the complex process of bringing this one product to market. In Virus and Cell Biology, the Hilleman teams had given way to Scolnick's research groups and to the new vaccine division headed by Gordon Douglas. Finally, in 1995, Merck's long-term investment began to pay off for the company, for the medical community, and for the children who were immunized.

Varivax would probably be one of the world's last attenuated, live-virus vaccines. The science and technology were changing rapidly, moving the industry in new directions. Recombinant DNA science and technology and new networks of private firms and public institutions were already launching the next long cycle of innovation as this one was ending. This transition was reflected at Merck in the changes that had taken place in Virus and Cell Biology since the mid-1980s.

During these same years, Merck was also bringing to completion what would probably be one of the last of the killed-virus vaccines, a defense against hepatitis A. Unlike hepatitis B, hepatitis A is transmitted orally and never develops into chronic liver disease. While usually a mild disease in children, hepatitis A can be severe in adults and is a particular problem in developing countries and among gay men.[70] A vaccine would be important not only to homosexual men, but also to travelers going from industrialized to developing countries,

---

69 When Dr. P. Roy Vagelos retired in November 1994, the Merck Board selected Raymond V. Gilmartin as the company's new chairman. Gilmartin had served as President and CEO since June of that year. An engineer by training, with an MBA from Harvard University, the fifty-three-year-old Gilmartin had previously been CEO and chairman of Becton Dickinson, a leading medical supply company. Under his leadership, Becton Dickinson had experienced substantial growth and expansion into global markets. Gilmartin was recognized in the industry as a business strategist with long-term vision and as an experienced leader in business-government relations.

70 F. Deinhardt and M. R. Hilleman, "Hepatitis A Vaccine," in Plotkin and Mortimer, eds., *Vaccines*, pp. 549–57. See also S. Krugman and R. Ward, "Clinical and Experimental Studies of Infectious Hepatitis," *Pediatrics* 22 (1958): 1016–22.

military personnel, institutionalized persons, children and employees in child-care centers, and healthcare workers.[71]

Hilleman had begun work on hepatitis A (HAV) before he left Walter Reed in the late 1950s, and at Merck, he and his coworkers had continued to struggle for some years with the problem of propagating HAV.[72] They finally began to make some progress after they adopted a marmoset model and established an epidemiological field study in San Jose, Costa Rica, under the direction of Dr. Victor M. Villarejos. Villarejos provided Virus and Cell Biology with the hepatitis specimens and data needed to continue this line of research in the 1970s.[73]

After another decade of research, Merck's project had completed a substantial amount of scientific groundwork on HAV, but it was 1979 before Hilleman and his colleagues had a vaccine within reach.[74] That year, they reported successful propagation of hepatitis A virus in cell culture.[75] This opened the way for Virus and Cell Biology

---

71 *New England Journal of Medicine* 327, no. 7 (1992): 488–90. *Lancet* (July 8, 1989): 114; (May 16, 1992): 1199; (July 25, 1992): 244.

72 This virus – like hepatitis B virus – could not be grown in vitro.

73 P. J. Provost, O. L. Ittensohn, V. M. Villarejos, J. A. Arguedas G., and M. R. Hilleman, "Etiologic Relationship of Marmoset-Propagated CR326 Hepatitis A Virus to Hepatitis in Man," *Proceedings of the Society for Experimental Biology and Medicine* 142 (1973): 1257–67. M. R. Hilleman, "Notes," MA.

74 Ibid.; see also pp. 276–82; ibid., 148 (1975): 532–9, 962–9; 155 (1977): 283–6; 159 (1978): 201–3. M. R. Hilleman, P. J. Provost, W. J. Miller, V. M. Villarejos, O. L. Ittensohn, and W. J. McAleer, "Development and Utilization of Complement-Fixation and Immune Adherence Tests for Human Hepatitis A Virus and Antibody," *American Journal of the Medical Sciences* 270, no. 1 (1975): 93–8. They presented other studies at the International Symposium on Viral Hepatitis in Milan in 1974 (*Developments in Biological Standardization* 30 [1975]: 383–9, 418–24). In addition to characterizing HAV as an enterovirus-like agent, they developed in vitro diagnostic assays, defined the seroepidemiology of hepatitis A, and provided proof of principle for a killed- or an attenuated-virus vaccine. See also *JAMA* 226, no. 13 (1973): 1507–8.

75 P. J. Provost and M. R. Hilleman, "Propagation of Human Hepatitis A Virus in Cell Culture in Vitro," *Proceedings of the Society for Experimental Biology and*

to develop either a killed- or attenuated-virus vaccine. Initially, they tried the latter path, with some success.[76] But following the transition in R & D leadership at Merck, Scolnick decided that the most promising approach would be with a killed-virus vaccine.[77] As the initial clinical studies indicated, the purified, formalin-inactivated vaccine was safe and immunogenic in healthy humans, and by 1991, the new research team had established the efficacy of a single shot of its new vaccine in a large, controlled trial.[78]

While the FDA was moving toward approval of Merck's *Vaqta*, the agency licensed a competing product from SmithKline Beecham

Medicine 160 (1979): 213–21. *New England Journal of Medicine* 327, no. 7 (1992): 489, called this a "giant step forward" in the search for a vaccine.

76 P. J. Provost, P. A. Giesa, W. J. McAleer, and M. R. Hilleman, "Isolation of Hepatitis A Virus *in Vitro* in Cell Culture Directly from Human Specimens," *Proceedings of the Society for Experimental Biology and Medicine* 167 (1981): 201–6. P. J. Provost, F. S. Banker, P. A. Giesa, W. J. McAleer, E. B. Buynak, and M. R. Hilleman, "Progress Toward a Live, Attenuated Human Hepatitis A Vaccine," in *Proceedings of the Society for Experimental Biology and Medicine* 170 (1982): 8–14. See also *Proceedings of the Society for Experimental Biology and Medicine* 172 (1983): 357– 63; M. R. Hilleman, P. J. Provost, E. B. Buynak, and A. A. McLean, "Progress Toward a Live Attenuated Human Hepatitis A Virus Vaccine," *Developments in Biological Standardization* 54 (1983): 433–40; and P. J. Provost, E. B. Buynak, A. A. McLean, M. R. Hilleman, and E. M. Scolnick, "Progress Toward a Live Attenuated Human Hepatitis A Vaccine," in Vyas, Dienstag, and Hoofnagle, eds., *Viral Hepatitis and Liver Disease*, pp. 467–75. The advantage of the attenuated live-virus over the inactivated-virus vaccine was that it would probably provide more lasting immunity. S. M. Lemon, "Type A Viral Hepatitis," *New England Journal of Medicine* 313, no. 17 (1985): 1059–67.

77 There were concerns about the safety and the stability of the live-virus product. See Lemon, "Type A Viral Hepatitis," pp. 1059–67, and *New England Journal of Medicine* 327, no. 7 (1992): 489.

78 A. Werzberger, B. Mensch, B. Kuter, L. Brown, J. Lewis, R. Sitrin, W. Miller, D. Shouval, B. Wiens, G. Calandra, J. Ryan, P. Provost, and D. Nalin, "A Controlled Trial of a Formalin-Inactivated Hepatitis A Vaccine in Healthy Children," *New England Journal of Medicine* 327, no. 7 (1992): 453–7; see also pp. 488–90. See also *Progress in Medical Virology* 37 (1990): 56–71.

Biologicals. SmithKline, which had already been marketing its vaccine in Europe for several years, also worked on a recombinant DNA product. But in this case the new technology was unsuccessful, and the killed-virus vaccines will be the standard product for immunization in the United States and abroad.[79] For Merck's vaccine division and for Virus and Cell Biology Research, *Vaqta* will be a significant and long-anticipated addition to the firm's list of vaccines.[80] It will not have the economic impact of the pediatric vaccines. But it will offer an important preventive measure to certain high-risk populations and especially to the growing number of international travelers flying between the developed and developing countries.

Unfortunately, neither Merck nor the researchers in other private and public laboratories have to date met with similar success in developing a vaccine against acquired immunodeficiency syndrome (AIDS).[81] Merck dedicated extensive resources to the search for an effective means of stopping an AIDS pandemic that is still spreading unchecked in the United States and many other countries around the world. The firm is continuing to make heavy investments in AIDS research and is currently testing a promising protease inhibitor. But the search for a vaccine continues to be hindered by "the worst possible confluence of viral and pathogenetic factors."[82]

---

79 See *JAMA* 267, no. 15 (1992); 271, no. 17 (1994), 1328–34, 1363–4. *Lancet* (May 16, 1992): 1198–9. *Wall Street Journal*, Aug. 13, 1992. *New York Times*, Aug. 13, 1992.

80 *Bulletin of the World Health Organization* 73, no. 1 (1995): 15–20.

81 *Military Medicine* 155, no. 6 (1990): 281–3.

82 M. R. Hilleman, "Conclusions: In Pursuit of an AIDS Virus Vaccine," in Jay A. Levy, ed., *AIDS: Pathogenesis and Treatment* (New York, 1988), pp. 609–11. Hilleman listed the following special problems: (1) the infection is transmitted by infected cells as well as free virus; (2) the viral DNA is integrated into the cell genome; (3) there is cell-to-cell transfer of the infection; (4) the virus is sequestered in the central nervous system; (5) there are numerous antigenic subtypes; (6) the virus impairs or destroys the immune system; and (7) there is no successful prototype lentivirus vaccine. See also M. R. Hilleman, "Perspectives in the Quest

While the current outlook is bleak, a similar prognosis could have been advanced about hepatitis A or B in the 1960s. Recent developments in science and technology are generating important opportunities to improve existing vaccines and to develop entirely new defenses against threatening infections. Those firms that have acquired and maintained capabilities in vaccine research, development, manufacturing, and marketing seem now to be poised on the edge of another long cycle of innovation.

In an effort to take full advantage of these opportunities, Merck completely reorganized its vaccine operations in 1994. To speed its decision making, the firm created a new unit that cut across divisional – that is, functional – lines and coordinated all research, production, and marketing for the vaccine business. This was the first such group that Merck has organized along strictly therapeutic lines. In this case, the organizational innovation reflected top management's confidence that the new scientific and technological networks relevant to vaccines were likely to remain unusually creative for many years to come. If they do and if the past is a fair guide to the future, Merck and the other leading companies in this industry will in the decades ahead provide us with protection against AIDS and the other new infections we will inevitably encounter.

---

for a Vaccine Against AIDS," in Dani Bolognesi, ed., *Human Retroviruses, Cancer, and AIDS* (New York, 1988), pp. 291–311. J. Cohen, "AIDS Vaccines: Are Researchers Racing Toward Success, or Crawling?" *Science* 265 (Sept. 2, 1994): 1373–5. Merck had by this time spent more than $359 million on AIDS research (both on vaccines and on drugs for treatment). R. G. Douglas, Jr., "The Implications of AIDS for the Development of Therapies and Vaccines: A Pharmaceutical Industry Perspective," in Caroline Hannaway, Victoria A. Harden, and John Parascandola, eds., *AIDS and the Public Debate* (Amsterdam, 1995), pp. 86–97.

CHAPTER 10

HISTORICAL PERSPECTIVES ON THE PROCESS OF INNOVATION

W
HAT, THEN, does an historical perspective help us understand about the process of innovation in modern, science-based industries? First, we believe, it enables us to see more clearly the pattern of long cycles that characterizes this process. In the case of vaccines and antitoxins, there have been four long cycles in the past century: the original, bacteriology cycle, which began in the late nineteenth century and sustained innovation in biologicals into the 1920s; the virology cycle, which developed in the 1940s and 1950s and exerted a dramatic influence on innovation through the 1960s, the 1970s, and into the 1980s; a third, less prominent long cycle in the 1960s and 1970s associated with the new bacteriology of polysaccharide capsules; and a fourth, more prominent long cycle – grounded in recombinant DNA technology and the new molecular understanding of genetics – beginning in the late 1970s and exerting a major influence on innovation in the 1980s and 1990s.

The development of organizational capabilities followed a similar pattern, as the companies sought to develop capacities for innovation suited to the networks and related sciences and technologies of their respective eras. At the level of the network, the long cycles were a function of the basic nature of scientific and technical paradigms, which have a tendency to yield diminishing commercial opportunities over time.[1] At

---

1 The periodization of these cycles was highly irregular; some were very long and the front across which innovation took place was in some cases extremely broad.

---

the level of the firm, the long cycles were in part normal organizational phenomena of the sort explored in the sociology of bureaucracy.[2] In the cases of Mulford, Sharp & Dohme, and Merck, each of the organizations had to acquire technical leadership of a relatively high quality to enable the company to understand and use the appropriate network information.[3] The research leaders within the firm had also to provide appropriate organizations for the discovery and development of the new products. They had an important role in production, especially during the initial stages of innovation. During the second long cycle, the one associated primarily with virology, the researchers at Merck — especially Maurice R. Hilleman — began to make important contributions to the science, as well as the technology, of vaccines.

Business management had primary responsibility for the related innovations in distribution, marketing, and finance; they were also responsible for the crucial decisions required if a company needed to make the transition to a new cycle. These transitions were particularly important aspects of the evolution of business capabilities. By the time a transition took place, a successful organization's leadership, culture, and network links were well established and could be difficult to change. New research leadership, with strong backing from the top executives and research managers, was usually needed to break existing

---

Others were shorter and the front narrower. For a description and analysis of the national context in which the U.S. components of these networks evolved see D. C. Mowery and N. Rosenberg, "The U.S. National Innovation System," in Nelson, ed., *National Innovation Systems*, pp. 29–75.

2 These long cycles should be distinguished from product cycles; the latter are intrinsically narrower and normally shorter than the cycles of innovation we have described.

3 N. Rosenberg, "Why Do Firms Do Basic Research (With Their Own Money)?" *Research Policy* 19, no. 2 (1990): 165–74. R. Henderson and I. Cockburn, "Measuring Competence? Exploring Firm Effects in Pharmaceutical Research," *Strategic Management Journal* 15, special issue (1994): 63–84.

patterns and develop new network-related capabilities. Scholars in business policy and in economics have begun to take note of these important transitions, and our study indicates that business historians can make an important contribution to that line of analysis.[4] Particularly interesting in this regard was the manner in which Merck's investments in the emerging virology cycle began to pay off just as the long cycle of innovation associated with medicinal chemistry was coming to an end. This helped prevent the kind of downturn that frequently accompanies these formative transformations in an industry.[5]

During a formative transition to a new science or technology, a firm's capabilities in basic research also came into play. Executives who were or had been leaders in basic research – scientists and science managers like Vagelos and Scolnick at Merck – were able to read the signals coming from the appropriate science and medical networks and guide their organizations through this type of transition to the next long cycle.[6] Even with effective leadership, this kind of formative transformation was not easy for a company to make. Without strong leadership –

---

4 See, for instance, Gambardella, *Science and Innovation*; and the same author's "Competitive Advantages From In-House Scientific Research: The U.S. Pharmaceutical Industry in the 1980s," *Research Policy* 21, no. 5 (1992): 391–407. R. M. Henderson and K. B. Clark, "Architectural Innovation: The Reconfiguration of Existing Product Technologies and the Failure of Established Firms," *Administrative Science Quarterly* 35, no. 1 (1990): 9–30. R. S. Rosenbloom and M. Christensen, "Technological Discontinuities, Organizational Capabilities, and Strategic Commitments," *Industrial and Corporate Change* 3, no. 3 (1994): 655–85.

5 On formative as opposed to adaptive or incremental change see L. Galambos, "The Innovative Organization: Viewed From the Shoulders of Schumpeter, Chandler, Lazonick, et al.," *Business and Economic History* 22, no. 1 (1993): 79–91.

6 Rosenberg, "Why Do Firms Do Basic Research (With Their Own Money)?" pp. 165–74, probes this issue from the perspective provided by economic theory. As Rosenberg concludes, "The performance of basic research may be thought of as a ticket of admission to an information network" (p. 170). See also Gambardella, "Competitive Advantages from In-House Scientific Research," pp. 391–407.

Mulford and Sharp & Dohme being cases in point — it was impossible to accomplish.

An historical perspective also helps us see how important markets, including the market for corporate control, were in shaping the patterns of innovation in this industry.[7] Active markets prompted the firms to accelerate and broaden the process of innovation. When capacities were underutilized — Mulford in the late 1920s; Sharp & Dohme in the early 1950s — the market for corporate control helped to move those resources into organizations that had the potential to use them more effectively. While Sharp & Dohme failed in this regard in the field of vaccines, Merck was remarkably successful and became one of ·the world's leading innovators in this important branch of preventive medicine.

The changing governmental context in the United States had an important impact on both the market for corporate control and the markets for vaccines. On the one hand, the federal government in the 1980s and 1990s relaxed the enforcement of the antitrust laws sufficiently to enable large firms like Merck either to acquire competitors or to establish alliances with other companies in this highly concentrated industry. Merck opted for the latter course, and the vaccine division created a number of important strategic alliances that broadened the front across which it innovates and enabled it to strengthen its position in global markets. On the other hand, one of the chief threats to the vaccine market in the post-World War II era was the tendency for national and international public-sector buying to narrow profit margins and drive firms out of the industry. From the 1970s on, oligopsony and monopsony linked with high liability risks made it difficult for companies like Merck to justify staying in the vaccine business on solely short-term economic grounds. By refusing

---

7 M. C. Jensen, "The Market for Corporate Control," in Newman, Milgate, and Eatwell, eds., *New Palgrave Dictionary of Money and Finance*, 2:657–66, describes recent developments.

to exit, however, Merck was able to position itself to take full advantage of the latest long cycle stemming from genetics and recombinant DNA technology.

These long cycles are, we believe, important aspects of innovative activity in all organizations, public or private. Our focus in this book has been primarily on the private sector. But the organizational processes we have examined have very general properties, and there is considerable evidence in secondary studies indicating that governmental and nonprofit institutions experience similar cycles of development. Scholars studying these organizations have not for the most part looked at them from this perspective, but we think this is a promising line of inquiry — one that would deepen our understanding of business-government relations as well as innovation. Especially important in this regard is the fact that public and nonprofit organizations respond primarily to nonmarket pressures and thus they experience the long cycles and the transitions in different ways than private-sector organizations.[8]

Not all of the developments we noted in the previous chapters were cyclical. There were significant linear changes as well. Over time the networks became more complex and differentiated, both internally and externally. The great expansion of scientific, medical, and technical institutions in the United States dramatically changed the manner in which firms in biologicals related to their environments. So too with the growth of the U.S. administrative state. The federal government became a regulator of economic activity and of all the enterprises in biologicals. In the years following World War II, the U.S. administra-

---

8 The effects may be unfortunate, making for inertia; public organizations respond more slowly and in less decisive ways to changes in their context than private corporations. But the effects may be favorable over the long term, as they were in the 1940s when the virology network continued to develop even though there was neither public support for it nor a market for innovative products like Squibb's pneumonia vaccine. See Chapter 3.

tive state also became a major promoter and subsidizer of scientific and medical research. Several of the most important innovative capabilities that firms had to develop were those related to the interfaces with government. Accomplishments in science and technology could easily be wiped out if a firm had unsatisfactory relations with the government. Over time, as U.S. firms expanded their global operations, they had to deal with a variety of political and administrative systems. As a result, political capabilities became an ever more significant aspect of innovation.

These changing contexts shaped the innovative activities of the three related firms we have examined. Their leaders had to devise strategies and business structures suited to these contexts, and above all, they had to acquire and support talented scientific and medical professionals who could provide dynamic R & D leadership within the firm and effective representation in the networks. As firm size grew, the firm's R & D leadership also had to compete for resources within the company and to maintain support for innovative processes extending over many years.

1

The H. K. Mulford Company had fewer of these problems to confront but resources that seem miniscule by the standards of the 1990s. Mulford was a tiny enterprise, resembling in some ways the start-up biotechnology firms of the 1980s and 1990s, except that these latter organizations have normally begun operations with considerable in-house technical and scientific talent. Initially, Mulford had to obtain even its scientific capability. It had very little capital. Its major advantages were a small, flexible organization, a sound entrepreneurial objective, and some solid experience in sales and marketing. Its major accomplishment was to promote aggressively the development of the new diphtheria serum antitoxin, to create an organization capable of fully exploiting the additional opportunities generated by the bacteriological revolution, and to organize a firm that could effectively distribute and market its innovative products. By World War I, it was one of the commercial leaders in the field of vaccines and antitoxins in the United States, with substantial standing overseas.

But as this long cycle drew to a close in the years following World War I, Mulford lost its innovative drive. What was lacking? In this instance, it was the general managerial capability to launch a new cycle of innovation. While it is true that diminishing returns were being experienced in the field of bacteriology, Mulford could have used its resources more creatively than it did. But like many family firms, its executives had expectational horizons bounded by their own careers, and as they neared retirement, they sold the company to an organization seeking to broaden its capabilities.

Sharp & Dohme's strategic plan was sound but its timing was terrible. The Great Depression undercut this initiative. But it is important to recognize that other firms in the industry – including Merck and Eli Lilly – were at this same time building the modern R & D organizations that would make them leaders in pharmaceutical innovation in the years to come. Sharp & Dohme attempted to follow their lead and certainly upgraded its research operations in the late 1930s and 1940s. But the company failed to build on the Mulford base it had purchased. Even when it had an unusual opportunity with its government-subsidized influenza vaccine to move to the front of the field in virology, the firm's leaders failed to raise the level of their vaccine research operation past the threshhold required to be an effective participant in these emerging networks. That left Sharp & Dohme selling the products of the previous cycle and unprepared to take advantage of the new long cycle taking shape.

Once again, resources in vaccine development that were being underutilized were transferred to new and more vigorous leadership by dint of corporate acquisition. In this case, the biological operations were an incidental element in the Merck, Sharp & Dohme merger of 1953. That, as well as the problems of consummating the combination, explains the delay Merck experienced in building its capabilities for innovation in virology. The crucial catalyst of change for the Merck Sharp & Dohme Research Laboratories was the new leadership provided by a scientist/science manager/science diplomat who had the energy and talent to enable the company to exploit fully the opportunities provided by this long cycle. Maurice R. Hilleman led Merck to a position of leadership in vaccine innovation, production, and marketing in the United States.

Merck was the first of the three organizations examined in this book to have the resources, the science management, and the executive leadership needed to elaborate and broaden its capabilities – in effect extending the long cycle of innovation for this firm. Two critical developments were the successful turn to polysaccharide capsular vaccines in the 1970s and the more trying transition to recombinant DNA technology and science in the 1980s. The latter transition was particularly challenging because at this same time, Merck's Virus and Cell Biology organization was experiencing a dramatic change in leadership. When Hilleman retired and Edward M. Scolnick took his place, Merck was on the edge of losing its position of prominence in vaccine R & D.

Many organizations fail at this point to develop the skills, leadership, and organization they need to take advantage of a new cycle forming outside the company. One of the reasons Merck was successful in this instance was the quality of its executive leadership. Under CEOs John J. Horan and P. Roy Vagelos, Merck had continued aggressively to strengthen its capabilities in vaccines. In the late 1970s, Merck considered but rejected a proposal to leave the field of vaccines. Then, in the early 1980s, Vagelos appointed Scolnick with an eye to his leadership in the emerging science of molecular genetics. Later, Vagelos promoted the establishment of a separate vaccine division under Gordon Douglas, who now led the firm's new, external growth initiative. These strategic alliances further broadened Merck's innovative capabilities in R & D and in global marketing. The company backed up these initiatives with substantial investments in research and production facilities and in development personnel and has continued on this course under CEO Gilmartin. It was this kind of effort that was required to see a market leader through a fundamental transformation of the sort that characterized this latest long cycle in vaccines.[9]

2

The transition in the 1990s was complicated by the substantial political crisis in the United States over healthcare reform. Merck's new vaccine division was barely up and running before the 1992 election brought into office an administration that opted to use vaccines as the opening wedge for the changes it hoped to make in the entire domestic healthcare field. Further complicating Gordon Douglas's tasks as head of the division was the manner in which the Clinton Administration employed an antibusiness rhetoric to sell its new program. At the heart of the Clinton proposal was a significant shift in the mixed system – a system blending public, nonprofit, and profit-making institutions – that had characterized this important corner of American medicine for many years. The long-term goal of the Administration was to improve immunization rates by centralizing authority in the system at the national level and creating a broad, new entitlement.

Merck, along with a large number of professionals in medicine, public health, and research, opposed the Clinton program on two primary grounds: first, that it deployed funds where they were not needed and failed to address the delivery problems that had long kept immunization levels for preschool children below acceptable levels; second, that it would over the long-term weaken innovation in vaccines by changing decisively the market conditions confronted by private-sector organizations.

Our long-term, historical study suggests a third reason to oppose a basic change in America's mixed, tripartite system. The

---

9 R. R. Nelson, "Why Do Firms Differ, and How Does It Matter?" *Strategic Management Journal* 12, special issue (1991): 61–74, addresses these general issues.

complex networks that have fostered innovation in vaccines and antitoxins blend the competencies of public, private, and nonprofit institutions, all of which respond to somewhat different signals and experience the transitions we have studied in different ways. The private firms read a combination of scientific/technical and market signals; the professional institutions read scientific/technical signals and blend them with signals about their members' functional concerns;[10] the public institutions blend political signals from the electorate, interest groups, and governmental bureaucracies with information of a scientific, technical, and professional nature. The public interest in disease control is best served over the long term, we believe, by having all of those signals read and responded to by an innovative, mixed system.[11]

As the Clinton plan moved into the legislature, its business and professional opponents picked up support from partisan political critics of the Administration and its fundamental approach to healthcare reform. This combination of forces helped block the most extreme of the proposals. Congress nevertheless approved a compromise version of the plan, only to learn in a few years from the General Accounting Office that the program's critics had been right.

Despite this vindication, the industry's political future seems far less secure than its economic, scientific, and technical prospects. As our historical study indicates, the mixed system in vaccines is inherently fragile and vulnerable to political attack. This is true even though on economic grounds the case for preventive medicine is irrefutable. As the efforts to rein in healthcare costs gather steam, the demand for vaccines and other preventive medicines will steadily increase. The demand will always be there – as the AIDS pandemic and the Ebola scare have made evident. On the supply side, the scientific and technical opportunities for vaccine development have never been richer than they are today. Companies like Merck and its three, major

---

10 These functional concerns normally have an important market component, but the markets are different from those confronting the private firms.

11 See also Nelson, "Why Do Firms Differ, and How Does It Matter?" p. 69.

global competitors have the capabilities to continue to discover, develop, produce, and distribute the innovative vaccine products the world needs. We will all be the poorer if through inadvertence or design we destroy any of the major participants in the complex networks of innovation that have evolved in the United States over the last, highly productive century.

ACKNOWLEDGMENTS

DHERING TO convention, we have placed our names on the title page of this book. Judging from that evidence alone, the book resulted from a joint effort by the team of Galambos and Sewell. But in reality this was a complex social enterprise that would have been impossible to complete without the support and assistance of a network of individuals and institutions. Now we get to thank them.

Heading the list is R. Gordon Douglas, Jr., President of Merck Vaccines. He sponsored the original project, was patient about our efforts to do additional research and to rewrite the manuscript for a university press, and gave the authors freedom to interpret the historical evidence our research uncovered. He had the support of many other persons at Merck, included two CEOs: first P. Roy Vagelos, M.D., and then Raymond V. Gilmartin. Edward M. Scolnick, M.D., Executive Vice President, Science and Technology, and President of the Merck Research Laboratories, gave us a helping hand, as did Senior Vice President and General Counsel, Mary M. McDonald, and the Vice President of Public Affairs, Kenneth C. Frazier. We are particularly grateful to Dr. Maurice R. Hilleman for the time he took to guide us toward additional sources and subjects of importance. His notes, oral history, and scientific publications were indispensable to our research.

Throughout the project, we received constant advice and support from Dr. Jeffrey L. Sturchio, who is an accomplished scholar as well as a Merck executive director. His administrative assistant, Patricia A. Fricke, and Eileen Carter were always helpful, as were the firm's archivists, Kabita Das and Debra Daniello. At several crucial points in the project, Catherine M. Maher brought her good judgment and intelligence to bear, helping us solve the problem of the day. Others at Merck who contributed in various ways are: Pamela Adkins, Albert D. Angel, Sharyn E. Bearse, Werten Bellamy, Richard C. Bostwick, William Ciacci, Jr., C. Boyd Clarke, Isabelle Claxton, Jean Lane Detwiler, Dr. Linda M. Distlerath, Dr. Stephen W. Drew, Frank Ecock, William H. Helfand, Lori F. Hirsch, C. Robin Hogen, Gary T. Kester, Marie H. Konarske, Linda J. Kratz, Kevin G. Lokay, Susan C. Mattson, Mary E. McAlpine, Brendan McNamara, Maureen D. Murphy, Ingrid Novak, Clyde Roche, Dr. Loren David Schultz, Dianne L. Snyder, Barbara J. Stass, William J. Vander Decker, Dr. Thomas M. Vernon, Jr., James W. Wallace, Louise F. Wisniewski, Johanna Wolski, and Christine M. Zettlemoyer.

At the Cambridge University Press, Frank Smith exceeded even his own fine record as an editor. His advice and support were invaluable; his efforts to bring the book out on schedule were astonishing – and successful. He was ably assisted by Alan Gold in production and by Waters Design Associates. Carol Bouyoucos of Waters designed the book, and we are grateful to Carol and to John Waters for making this volume attractive. Huron Valley Graphics did a fine job printing the book on a tight schedule, and we are especially grateful to Kevin M. Rennells for his help. Two anonymous readers for Cambridge provided a number of suggestions that enabled us to improve the manuscript as we approached publication.

There would not have been a manuscript without substantial assistance from Johns Hopkins University and from the Business History Group (BHG). Steve and Madeleine Adams provided invaluable help with the research, as did Dr. Patricia A. Watson. Madeleine Adams carried the project through to completion as a combined copyeditor/project manager. Nora Kay Moran helped launch the book phase of this undertaking. She did an excellent job of organizing the early research and keeping us on course, as did BHG's astute business manager, Bob Lewis. Lynn K. Gorchov brought her talents and experience to bear on our index, making the book considerably more useful to our readers. At Johns Hopkins, we had the support of the Department of the History of Science, Medicine, and Technology; in particular, we appreciate the contributions of Chair Gert H. Brieger, M.D., Harry M. Marks, Edward T. Morman, and Arthur Silverstein. In the Hopkins Department of History, we are especially grateful for the help we received from Sarah Springer, Shirley Hipley, and Sharon Widomski. Chairs Richard Goldthwaite and Dorothy Ross did their best to keep Hopkins the unique place that it is for scholarly research and writing.

So many colleagues in Hopkins, Merck, and elsewhere contributed ideas that we can only issue a blanket "thank you" covering our friends from all over the United States, Norway, the United Kingdom, Italy, and Holland. We thank them for reading draft chapters and for offering us their suggestions. They all helped to make this a better book.

A WORD ABOUT SOURCES

OUR FOOTNOTES are, we believe, the best guide to the sources used in writing this book. Full references to all of the articles appear in the first citation in any chapter. Full references to the books appear where they are cited for the first time in the volume. As the footnotes indicate, the bulk of the manuscript materials used in writing *Networks of Innovation* came from the archives of Merck & Co., Inc. The Merck Archives (MA), originally established by Dr. Jeffrey L. Sturchio in 1989 and now directed by Kabita Das, are located in Whitehouse Station, New Jersey, at Merck's international headquarters. All of the internal company materials — whether located there or elsewhere — were made available to us through the Merck Archives and are cited in that manner.

In Philadelphia, Pennsylvania, we located additional primary materials at two collections. The Library of the College of Physicians of Philadelphia (LCPP) has various assorted manuscripts and secondary studies related to Mulford, Sharp & Dohme, and Merck. These include early price lists and advertising for the H. K. Mulford Company and its various vaccines and antitoxins. The University of Pennsylvania Archives (UPA) — where we were kindly assisted by Archivist Gail M. Pietrzyk — has a large, well-organized collection of the papers of Dr. Alfred Newton Richards, who was for many years a scientific consultant to Merck. Richards became a member of Merck's Board of Directors in 1948 and chaired the Board's scientific committee from 1949 to

1956. These papers include important manuscripts pertaining to the Merck Institute for Therapeutic Research, as well as the firm's general research program.

We searched the Kremer Reference Files in the F. B. Power Pharmaceutical Library. The Library, which is part of the University of Wisconsin in Madison, has a good collection of manuscript and printed materials, particularly advertisements from the industry's leading firms.

In and around Washington, D.C., we found several public collections extremely useful. The Library of Congress (LC) has a large collection of the papers of Dr. Vannevar Bush, who joined the Merck Board of Directors in 1949 and then succeeded George W. Merck as chairman from 1957 to 1962. These materials include correspondence and minutes of committees on which Bush served. We also made considerable use of the records in the National Archives (NA), where Mrs. Aloha South guided us to the materials we needed. The staff at the National Records Center in Suitland, Maryland, was also helpful as we searched the Center's voluminous records. We found some materials relevant to vaccines and antitoxins at the History of Medicine Division of the National Library of Medicine in Bethesda, Maryland.

Because we focused on professional/corporate/public networks, the extensive collections at the Johns Hopkins University's Medical Institutions were indispensable to our research effort. We drew heavily on the library of the School of Hygiene and Public Health. We also did a substantial amount of research in the serials held in the Welch Institute for the History of Medicine and the Welch Library. They offer outstanding sources for any scholar interested in the history of modern medicine.

INDEX

AB Astra, 217
acne, 23
Aconite, 11 n8
acquired immunodeficiency syndrome (AIDS),
189, 195; pandemic of, 238, 250; research
on, 238–9; *see also* human
immunodeficiency virus (HIV)
Adams, John, 14
adenoviruses, 69, 127 n8; vaccine, 65
adjuvants, 135 n34, 136, 137 n40, 203
Adjuvant 65, 136, 137 n40, 138
Africa, 27, 112 n97, 119, 153 n7, 156, 163,
185
Agency for International Development (AID),
119, 220
Alberts, A. W., 83 n13
Alexander cells, 196–7
amantadine, 144 n58
American Academy of Arts and Sciences, 125
American Academy of Pediatrics (AAP), 116
n112, 171; Committee on Infectious Diseases, 172 n67
"American Century," 53, 55, 123, 209
American Chemical Society, 125
American Cyanamid, 213
American Home Products, 213 n4
American Hospital Association (AHA), 73 n53
American Medical Association (AMA), 73 n53,
75–6
ampicillin, 169
Amprol, 127 n7
analgesics, 145 n63
anthrax, 5; antitoxin, 21 n28, 22; vaccine, 21
n28, 39
antibiotics, 51; discovery of, 37; expectations

for, 37, 43, 50; for meningitis, 152, 169–
70; for pneumococcal pneumonia, 159–
60; produced by Merck, 56–7, 120, 145,
208; research and development of, 38; resistance to, 169
antibodies, *see by name of disease*
antigenic mass, 144 n58
antigenic potency of vaccines, 136 n36
antigenic relationships, 46
antigenic shift: in influenza, 66, 72–3, 132–3,
134–6, 137 n40; in swine influenza, 138
antigenic specificity, 72–3
antigens, 20, 22 n34, 23, 41; hepatitis, 186–
90, 193, 196–200, 202–4; HIB meningitis, 153, 173–4; influenza, 46–7, 72, 136
n37; measles, 91 n34; pneumonia, 159
antihypertensive drugs, 120
anti–infective drugs, 37, 56
anti–inflammatory drugs, 120, 145
antiparasitic drugs, 127 n7
antitoxins, 23, 211, 241, 247; abandonment
of, 37, 49–50; and coinage of word, 8;
distribution of, xi, 32; innovation in, ix–
xiii; licensing of, 21–2; marketing of, xiii,
18–20, 246; measles, 86; meningitis,
152; pneumonia, 39, 158–9; production
of, xi, xiii, 158–9; research and development of, ix, xi, xiii; standardization of,
18–9; streptococcic infection, 22, 24n, 33
n1; tetanus, 21, 22, 33 n1, 39; *see also*
diphtheria antitoxins; H. K. Mulford Company
antitrust laws, 217 n13, 244
antivaccination movement, 6
antiviral drugs, 84

259

antiviral screening, 84
Armed Forces Epidemiological Board, 73, 100 n60, 153
Armed Forces laboratories, 86
Armed Services, see military, U.S. Army, U.S. Navy
Aronson, Hans, 19 n25
Artenstein, Malcolm S., 106, 153
arthralgia, 113
arthritis, 113, 145
arthropathy, 113 n100, 215 n8
Asia, 53, 69, 123, 133, 185, 207–8, 219
Asian influenza, see influenza virus (Type A₂)
Attenuvax, 98, 117 n114
Australia, 28, 105, 112 n97, 185, 186, 219–20
Austrian, Robert, 157, 160–2, 166–8, 189, 232 n63
Avery, Oswald, 25, 159–60
avian leukosis (chicken leukemia), 94–5, 101, 128–9

bacteremia, 158, 170 n64
bacterial epiglottitis, 170 n64
bacterial meningitis, *see H. influenzae* Type B meningitis
bacterins: definition of, 159; and H. K. Mulford Company, 22–4, 39; and Sharp & Dohme Company, 159
bacteriology: frontier in, 42; innovation in, 3–4, 50, 241; networks, 157; of polysaccharide capsules, 241; research and development in, 2, 4–5, 7, 13–14, 16, 21 n28, 25, 152, 247; revolution, ix, 29, 211, 246
Baltimore Aircoil Company, 131 n20
Banyu (Japan), 58
Barclay, Eugene S., 73–4
Becton Dickinson, 235 n69
Behring, Emil von, 7, 8, 19
Behringwerke (Germany), 146, 173
Belgium, 112 n97, 146, 196n43, 205 n62
Belladonna, 11 n8
Biavax (mumps-rubella), 118
Biggs, Herman M., 15
biochemistry, 54, 83 n13, 84 n16, 124–6
biologicals, *see* antitoxins, blood products, diphtheria antitoxins, vaccines, *by name of vaccine*
Biologicals Control Act (1902), 22, 30 n54
Biologics Control Laboratory, 61 n20, 73 n55; *see also* Division of Biologics Standards (DBS), Food and Drug Administration
biosynthesis, 125, 200

biotechnology: companies, 199, 246; research at Merck, xi, 200, 202, 230; *see also* genetic engineering, genetics, recombinant DNA technology
Birnbaum, Jerome, 198
birth defects: from measles, 104; from mumps, 99, 104; from rubella, 104–5, 106–7
black-leg disease vaccine, 21 n28
Blake, Francis G., 39 n13
blood banks, 186
blood products, 39, 51, 190; *see also* gamma globulin, plasma
Blumberg, Baruch S., 186, 187 n18, 188
Bodian, David, 60 n16
Brazil, 155–6
bronchopulmonary infections, 170 n64
brucellosis: antitoxin, 22; vaccine, 41
Buescher, E. L., 106
Bumpers, Dale, 228, 229 n51
Bureau of Biologics (BoB), *see* Food and Drug Administration
Burmester, Benjamin R., 129
Burnet, Sir Macfarlane, 105
Burroughs, Wellcome & Company (United Kingdom), 23 n37, 119 n119, 146
Bush, George, 217 n13
Bush, Vannevar, 62–3, 68
Buynak, Eugene B., 101, 104, 107, 188 n22, 203 n58

Calgon Corporation, 131 n20
Campbell, Milton, 11, 13–14, 28
Canadian Public Health Service, 119
cancer, 82; in animals, 127–31; research, 129, 173 n70, 202 n54; as result of hepatitis, 185–6, 196–7; vaccine, 130–1; viral etiology of, 83, 130–1; *see also* avian leukosis, cervical cancer, liver cancer, sarcoma virus
Carlo, D. J., 162 n36
cellulitis, 170 n64
Centers for Disease Control (CDC), 42, 147; Advisory Committee on Immunization Practices (ACIP), 138–9, 166 n50, 172 n67; and healthcare reform, 228 n50, 229 n52; hepatitis unit (Phoenix, Arizona), 192 n34; and influenza, 73, 76; and measles, 116 n112; and pneumonia, 166 n50, 167 n53; and swine influenza, 138–9, 141
cervical cancer, 219 n20
Chandler, Alfred D., x, 9n
Charney, Jesse, 79
Chemo-Sero-Therapeutic Research Institute (Japan), 205 n62, 219

261

138; bivalent (Type A plus Type B) killed-virus, 48; clinical testing of, 132, 135–7, 167; controversy about, 132–3; distribution of, 75, 76 n62, 134; killed-virus, 48, 134, 144; licensing of, 133–4; markets for, 132, 144; and the military, 41, 43–5, 47–8, 69, 75; monovalent (A$_2$), 75; polyvalent (A, A$_1$, and B), 74, 134; production of, 41, 47–8, 73–6, 132, 134, 139; public pressure for, 75–6; reactions to, 136, 143; reactogenicity of, 49, 90; research and development of, 46–8, 71–2, 134–6, 197; sales of, 49; for Type A influenza virus, 46, 72; for Type A$_2$ (Hong Kong) influenza virus, 73–5, 133–4, 137; for Type B influenza virus, 46, 132; see also Adjuvant 65

influenza viruses: antigenic relationship to swine influenza, 46; antigenic shift and drift in, 66, 72–3, 132–3, 134–6, 137 n40; antigenic specificity of, 72–3; research on, 46–8, 70, 71–4; Type A, 46–7, 72, 132, 144 n58; Type A$_1$, 72; Type A$_2$ (Hong Kong), 72–4, 133–4, 137, 144 n58; Type B, 46–7, 132; Type C, 46 n26

Institute of Medicine, 184, 225–6; Committee on Public-Private Sector Relations in Vaccine Innovation, 177–8

Institut Mérieux (France), 155 n15, 213

International Center for Medical Research and Training (San Jose, Costa Rica), 112 n95

international organizations, x, 218 n15; and immunization campaigns, 55–6, 119, 205–7, 220–1; see also Pan American Health Organization, Project HOPE, UNICEF, World Bank Group, World Health Organization

Intervet International (Netherlands), 200 n51

Investigative New Drug (IND) Regulations, 162 n38

Japan, 58, 232; influenza in, 72, 74, 133; market for vaccines in, 216; vaccine producers in, 194 n40, 205 n62

Japanese B encephalitis vaccine, 69

jaundice, yellow, 183, 184 n7, 185; see also hepatitis

Jenner, Edward, 5–6

Johnson, C. D., 100

Johnson & Johnson, 217

Johnson, Lyndon Baines, 63 n25, 107, 123

joint ventures, see strategic alliances

Juselius Foundation, Sigrid, 154 n11

Kalabus, F., 119

Katz, Samuel, 87

Kefauver-Harris Drug Amendment Act of 1962, 131 n19, 222

Kelco Company, 131 n20

kidney disease, 158

Kimber Farms, 95

Kinyoun, Joseph James, 25

Kitasato, Shibasaburo, 8

Koch, Robert, 4, 7, 18; Institute (Germany), 15; postulates of, 4n, 127

Koop, C. Everett, 226 n41

Korea Green Cross Corporation, 219 n18

Korean War, 184

Krah, David, 201

Krugman, Saul, 88, 189–91, 192 n32

Lampson, George P., 188 n22

Lasker, Mary, 109

Lasker Foundation, Albert and Mary, 109

Latin America, 58, 155

Lederle Antitoxin Laboratories, 27 n46; as competitor in vaccine market, 23 n37, 146, 168 n56; production of vaccines by, 80 n4, 96 n50, 171 n67

Lederle Praxis Biologicals, 213

lentivirus vaccine, 238 n82

liability, 64, 178, 213, 224, 225–6 n36, 244; for influenza vaccines, 145; for measles vaccine, 91 n34; for pediatric vaccines, 61 n21, 178; for polio vaccines, 61–2, 80–3; for rubella vaccine, 110; for swine influenza vaccine, 142–3

licensing, foreign, 112, 138, 204

licensing, U.S. government, 147, 173; of adjuvants, 138; of antitoxins, 21–2; of chicken pox vaccine, 234; of combination vaccines, 97, 118, 174–5; of hepatitis globulin, 187; of hepatitis vaccines, 193, 204, 237–8; of HIB meningitis vaccine, 174–5; of influenza treatments, 144 n58; of influenza vaccines, 48, 133–4, 138; of measles vaccines, 91 n34, 96–7, 115, 119; of meningitis vaccines, 152, 155, 156; of mumps vaccine, 103; of pneumonia vaccines, 37, 164; of polysaccharide capsular vaccines (PRP), 171; of rubella vaccine, 112, 114 n101; of veterinary vaccines, 130, 147

Lilly & Company, Eli, 173 n70; abandonment of vaccine research by, 146, 161, 183; as competitor in pharmaceutical market, 35, 247; production of vaccines by, 96 n50

Lincoln, Clarence W., 14, 25

121, 131, 247; organizational capabilities of, x–xi, 84 n16, 181–2, 212, 241–3, 247–8; patent protection and, 124, 186 n17, 213–14; pharmaceutical research and development by, 56–8, 70, 83 n13, 120, 124–6, 140, 145, 152, 208, 210; sales of, 57, 96, 114, 115, 119 n119, 120, 124, 146, 147; standardization at, 140–1; strategic alliances of, 217–19, 244, 248; strategy of, 58, 63, 76, 124, 131 n19, 205, 210, 214, 217–18; subsidiaries of, 58, 131, 219; and university cooperation, 17n, 84–5, 88–93, 97–8, 101–2, 107–12, 118, 134–6, 161–8, 189–92, 198–200, 232; and U.S. government relations, xi, 61, 73–6, 107, 131, 133–4, 138–43, 147–8, 154, 162 n38, 164 n44, 176–9, 222–9, 244–6, 249; and virology program of, 60, 62, 63 n26, 79–80, 84, 96, 152, 176; *see also* licensing-foreign, licensing-U.S. government, Merck Institute for Therapeutic Research, Merck Sharp & Dohme Research Laboratories, Merck Virus and Cell Biology Research

Merck Institute for Therapeutic Research, 64 n27, 71, 83, 100, 178–9; Division of Virus and Tissue Culture Research (West Point, Pennsylvania), 58, 60,A 64, 71, 79, 83, 93, 97, 136 n37, 162; *see also* Merck Virus and Cell Biology Research

Merck Sharp & Dohme (MSD), 71, 126 n6; foreign branches of, 154–5 n12; marketing by, 115, 216; sales growth of, 121

Merck Sharp & Dohme International (MSDI), 146–7, 216

Merck Sharp & Dohme Research Laboratories (MSDRL), 71; Biological Process Improvement Laboratories, 97; Biological Production Division (West Point, Pennsylvania), 73, 140, 141, 210, 215, 230; Division of Toxicology and Pathology, 93; formation of, 56–8; Glenolden biological operations of, 58; leadership in, 57, 58, 60–1, 62, 63 n26, 84 n16, 125–7, 145, 151, 181–3, 208–9; Veterinary Department, 93; *see also* Merck & Co., Inc, Merck Institute for Therapeutic Research, Merck Virus and Cell Biology Research, *by name of disease, by name of vaccine*

Merck Vaccine Division, x, xii, 218

Merck *Vaccine Study – 1979*, 145–9, 151, 157, 213

Merck Virus and Cell Biology Research: innovation in, 103, 121, 147, 151–2, 176, 181–2, 198, 210; institutional transition to biotechnology in, 126, 197–99, 200–2, 204 n61, 208–10, 235, 243–4, 248–9; leadership in, 71–2, 76–77, 176, 200–2, 210, 243–4, 247–8; *see also* Merck & Co., Inc., Merck Institute for Therapeutic Research, Merck Sharp & Dohme Research Laboratories, *by name of disease, by name of vaccine*

Mérieux (France), 146, 219

Mérieux/Connaught, 217

Meriweather, Delano, 143

Merrell-National Laboratories, 140, 155 n14, 157 n20

Meruvax, 112, 114–15, 117

metabolic disease, 158

Metalsalts Corporation, 131 n20

Metchnikoff, Elie, 7

Mevacor (lovastatin), 83 n13, 208

Meyer, Jr., Harry, 109, 110 n90, 111, 119

Milanovic, Milan, 87

military, 69 n39, 154 n12; influenza in, 41, 43–5, 47–8, 69, 75; outbreaks of disease in, 106, 138, 153–4, 183–4, 235–6; and plasma, 39–41; and purchase of antitoxins by, 27; purchase of vaccines by, 41, 75, 154; research on diseases in, 65–6, 106; research on vaccines in, 47–8, 69–70, 86–7, 153; swine influenza in, 138–9

Miller, William J., 203 n58

Millman, Irving, 186 n17

Minnesota, 25 n40, 228 n49

M-M-R (measles-mumps-rubella), 118, 127

M-M-R II (measles-mumps-rubella), 215–16

M-M-Vax (measles-mumps), 118

Molitor, Hans, 71

M-R-Vax (measles-rubella), 118

MSD, *see* Merck Sharp & Dohme

MSDRL, *see* Merck Sharp & Dohme Research Laboratories

Mulford, Henry K., 10–11, 13–14, 28

Mulford Company, H. K., 4, 160 n30; and antitoxins (in general), x, 21, 22–4, 28, 37, 39, 86, 152, 158; assets of, 11, 14; and biologicals; 3, 10 n2, 18, 21, 22 n33, 25, 27, 28, 211; Board of Directors of, 14; branch offices of, 11, 27; and competition, 9, 30–1; and diphtheria antitoxins, 7–8, 9, 13–22, 26, 28, 246–7; distribution by, 3, 25, 27–8, 32, 246;

Mulford Company, H. K. (*cont.*)
entrepreneurial efforts by, 7, 10–1, 17, 28–9, 30, 246; Glenolden Biological Laboratories of, 18–9, 24, 27; growth of, 24–5, 27; and innovation, ix–xii, 13, 17, 19, 21 n29, 28–30, 43, 55, 247; leadership in, 10–1, 29–30, 242, 244; and licensing, 21–2; marketing by, 18–20, 31 n56, 246; merger with Sharp & Dohme, x, xiii, 28, 33–4, 38, 50, 158, 247; organizational capabilities of, x, 9, 241–3; origins of, 10–1; production by, 10–1, 14–19, 24–5, 26, 28, 31, 37, 97 n53; products of, 3, 10–11, 17, 21–3, 24n, 26–8, 32, 39; and public health network, 3, 15–16; and regulation, 30–2; research and development by, x, 13–17, 21, 23–4, 25–6, 28–9, 31, 39; sales of, 11, 17, 19, 21, 22, 25, 28; staff of, 18, 25, 27; standardization by, 18–19, 31; and university-industry cooperation, 16–18; and U.S. government relations, 15–16, 27, 30–2; and vaccines, x, 18, 21–3, 25 n42, 26 n43, 28, 39, 97 n53, 247
multinational corporations, 53, 55, 131
mumps, 106; antibodies to, 100–3, 107–9; complications of, 99–100, 104; epidemics of, 102, 103 n70; immmunization for, 102 n66, 115–16; incidence of, 90, 116; *Jeryl Lynn* virus strain of, 100–1, 118; research on, 100–1
mumps vaccines: clinical testing of, 100, 101–3, 111; combination, 117–20, 215–6, 230 n54; efficacy of, 102; innovation in, 127; killed-virus, 100; licensing of, 103; live-virus, 100–2; production of, 101 n62; research and development of, 100–1, 152, 188; sales of, 115–16, 120; *see also* Mumpsvax
Mumpsvax, 103, 115–16, 117
municipal health agencies, *see* public health
Murray, R., 81 n7

Nashville, Tennessee: HIB meningitis study in, 170
National Academy of Sciences, 125
National Cancer Institute: Genetics Section, 173 n70
National Childhood Vaccine Injury Act, 61 n21, 178
National Foundation for Infantile Paralysis, 74 n57; Technical Committee, 59
National Heart Institute, 125 n4, 173 n70

National Immunization Program, 139–43, 147; *see also* swine influenza
National Institute of Allergy and Infectious Diseases (NIAID), 138 n43, 148, 218; and clinical testing of vaccines, 112, 164 n44; and research on vaccines, 154 n11, 160–1, 197 n46; Vaccine Development Board of, 109
National Institute of Child Health and Human Development, 168
National Institutes of Health, 125 n4, 148, 202 n54; and influenza vaccine, 73–4, 75; and polio vaccine, 81–2; support of research by, 42, 212 n3; Task Force on Tissue Culture Viruses and Vaccines, 83 n12; Technical Committee, 81 n7; *see also* Biologics Control Laboratory, Division of Biologics Standards (DBS), Food and Drug Administration
National Vaccine and Antitoxin Institute, 23 n37
Native Americans, 161, 174, 227
Neff, Beverly Jean, 104
Netherlands Red Cross Blood Transfusion Service, 193 n35
New Jersey Department of Health, 138 n43
New York Blood Center, 186 n17, 192
New York City, 19, 33, 192; pharmaceutical industry in, 9–10
New York City Health Department: and diphtheria antitoxins, 7–8, 13, 14, 15–16; Division of Pathology, Bacteriology, and Disinfection, 2, 7–8, 10; and smallpox vaccination, 6–7
New York City Metropolitan Board of Health: origins of, 2; replacement by New York City Health Department, 6 n14; research by, 2, 14; *see also* New York City Health Department
New York University College of Medicine, 189–90
Nicrazan, 127 n7
Nollstadt, K., 162 n36

Office of Naval Research, 63 n25
Office of Scientific Research and Development (Washington, D.C.), 63 n25, 68
oncology studies, 83
opsonins, 24
organizational capabilities: of Merck, x–xi, 84 n16, 181–2, 212, 241–3, 247–8; of Mulford, x, 9, 241–3; of Sharp & Dohme, x, 34, 50, 241–3

respiratory diseases, 161; *see also* adenoviruses
respiratory syncytial virus (RSV), 177, 181
    n1
retroviruses, 130
Reyes v. Wyeth (1974), 142 n54
Rhone-Poulenc, S. A., 213 n5
Richards, Alfred Newton, 63
Richardson-Merrell, 146
RIT (Belgium and Holland), 146
river blindness (onchocerciasis), 207; *see also*
    Mectizan
Rockefeller Foundation, 220
Rockefeller Institute (New York), 25 n42, 46,
    184 n7
Rockefeller Institute for Comparative Physiol-
    ogy (Princeton), 45
Rocky Mountain Spotted Fever, 39 n11; vac-
    cine, 39
Roehm, Robert E., 188 n22
Romania, 220–1
Roux, Emil, 8, 19 n25
rubella (German measles): antibodies to, 105,
    111, 113; Benoit strain of, 107–8; compli-
    cations of, 104–5, 106, 108; epidemics of,
    106–7, 110, 114; etiology of, 106 n76;
    HPV-77 strain of, 109–10, 113, 118; im-
    munization for, 110, 112, 113–14; inci-
    dence of, 114; and morbidity, 104 n72;
    and mortality, 104 n72; outbreaks of, 104,
    106, 111; public health campaigns for,
    114; RA 27/3 strain of, 113 n100, 117
    n114, 215; reactogenicity of, 112–13; re-
    search on, 105–6, 107
rubella vaccine: clinical trials of, 109, 110–14,
    120 n123; combination, 117–20, 215–
    16, 230 n54; efficacy of, 110, 111; HPV-
    77 duck embryo, 118; innovation in,
    127; international conference on, 112;
    killed-virus, 107–8; liability of, 110; li-
    censing of, 112, 114 n101; live-virus,
    108–14; production of, 112; public de-
    mand for, 106–7; reactions to, 113; re-
    actogenicity of, 112–13; research and de-
    velopment of, 103, 105–10, 111 n92,
    152, 188, 215; sales of, 114 n103; *See*
    also Meruvax
Rubeovax, 96–7, 101 n62, 115, 119, 128
Rubin, Harry, 95
Rutter, William, 198–200
Sabin, Albert, 69 n39, 80 n4; vaccine of, 80,
    83 n12, 142 n54
saccharomyces cervisiae; see yeast
Salk, Jonas, 47, 64 n27, 83 n12; vaccine of,

59, 60 n16, 61 n20, 62 n22, 64, 73 n55,
    79–83
sarcoma virus, 173 n70
Sayre, Lucius P., 10
scarlet fever, 86 n22
Schaffner, William, 233 n63
Schultz, Loren D., 202 n54
Schumpeter, Joseph A., 229 n53
Sclavo (Italy), 146
Scolnick, Edward M., as leader of Merck Virus
    and Cell Biology Research, 172–3, 174
    n72, 182 n3, 200–2, 204 n61, 210, 235,
    237, 243, 248; as president of Merck
    Sharp & Dohme Research Laboratories,
    182, 191, 210; training of, 173 n70
Sell, Sarah W., 170–1
septic arthritis, 170 n64
serobacterins, 22–3, 24n, 39; definition of, 159
seroconversion, 204 n59
serological response, 136, 192
serological testing, 186
serotypes of HIB, 169–70; of influenza virus,
    46–7; of meningococcus, 153–4, 156
    n18; of pneumonococcus, 37, 158–9, 160
    n30, 162–5; of poliomyelitis virus, 59, 79
serum antitoxins, *see* antitoxins
serum hepatitis, *see* hepatitis B
sexually transmitted diseases: development of
    vaccine for, 219–20 n20
Shalala, Donna E., 227, 228
Sharp & Dohme (S & D): and antitoxins, x, 33
    n1, 35, 39, 51; and biologicals, 33–4,
    38–9, 42–3, 48, 50–1, 158–9; Board of
    Directors of, 34; branch offices of, 33; and
    competition, 34, 35; distribution by, 33,
    39, 58; growth of, 38; and innovation, ix–
    xii, 37–43, 48, 50–1; leadership in, 34–
    5, 43, 51, 57, 242, 244, 247; and licens-
    ing, 48; marketing by, 34, 50; merger
    with Merck & Company, Inc., x, xiii, 28,
    38, 51, 56–7, 64 n27, 71, 121; merger
    with H. K. Mulford Company, x, xiii, 28,
    33–4, 38, 50, 158, 247; Mulford Biologi-
    cal Laboratories (Glenolden, Pennsylvania)
    of, 34, 38–41, 50, 159; organizational ca-
    pabilities of, x, 34, 50, 241–3; origins of,
    33; and pharmaceuticals, 35 n6; produc-
    tion by, 33–4, 35 n6, 39, 47–8, 97 n53,
    158–9; products of, 33–5, 39 n11, 45,
    50, 51, 57; reorganization of, 33–4; re-
    search and development by, x, 33–5, 37–
    8, 42, 48, 50–1, 54, 158–9, 247; sales
    of, 33 n1, 38; staff of, 35, 38; and U.S.

network, 138 n43; *see also* military, Walter Reed Army Institute of Research, Walter Reed Army Graduate School

U.S. Army Epidemiological Board, 47; Commission on Neurotropic Virus Diseases, 69 n39

U.S. Army 406th Medical General Laboratory (Zamo, Japan), 72

U.S. Army special commission on influenza and other epidemics, *see* U.S. Army Epidemiological Board

U.S. Department of Agriculture, 128, 129; Regional Poultry Research Laboratory (East Lansing, Michigan), 129

U.S. Department of Health and Human Services, 148, 227, 228; Steering Committee for Development of a Health Research Strategy, 148

U.S. Department of Health, Education, and Welfare, 82, 139

U.S. government: and encouragement of generic vaccines, 147; immunization legislation of, 107; immunization policy of, 113–14, 223–9; immunization recommendations of, 103, 167, 171; and influenza epidemic, 45, 73–4; and meningitis, 153–4; and pressure for vaccine development, 61, 155; price controls, 131, 223; purchase of antitoxins and vaccines by, 27, 61, 74, 140, 154, 178, 213, 225–6, 228, 244; support for research, 54, 68, 123, 212; and swine influenza, 138–43; and vaccine innovation, 148, 177–8; and vaccine standards, 93; *see also* immunization, liability, licensing, Merck & Co. Inc., Mulford Company, National Immunization Program, regulation; Sharp & Dohme, *U.S. government organizations by name*

U.S. Navy, 154

U. S. Public Health Service, 173 n70; Advisory Committee on Immunization Practices, 103; and influenza, 73; (Washington) laboratory of, 25; origins of, 2 n4; reports of, 26 n43; and swine influenza, 139 n46; and vaccines, 80, 100, 101, 171; *see also* Centers for Disease Control, Marine Hospital Service; Public Health and Marine Hospital Service

United States Standard Serum Company, 27 n46

U.S. Surgeon General, 82, 133–4, 226 n41

U.S. Surgeon Inspector, 24n

University of California at Berkeley, 95, 198–9

University of Chicago, 67–9

University of Pennsylvania, 25, 123 n4; Laboratory of Hygiene, 13, 16–17, 18; Medical Department, 13; Veterinary School, 14, 18

University of Pennsylvania Hospital Pepper Clinical Laboratory, 13

University of Pennsylvania School of Medicine, 157; Department of Pediatrics, 85, 89, 97–8, 101, 118, 135, 232; *see also* Children's Hospital (Philadelphia)

University of Pittsburgh, 59

University of Washington, 199, 202 n54

vaccination, *see* immunization

vaccine industry, economic problems of, 145–6, 147–8

vaccines, *see by name of vaccine*

Vaccines for Children (VFC) program, 228–9

vaccinia virus, 97

vaccinus, definition of, 5

Vagelos, P. Roy: as CEO of Merck & Co., Inc., 178–9, 182–3, 208, 214, 218, 222–3, 227, 234–5, 248; as president of Merck Sharp & Dohme Research Laboratories (MSDRL), 125–7, 145, 197–8, 200, 204 n61, 243; research and training of, 125, 151

Valenzuela, Pablo, 198–9

Vanderbilt University Medical School, 170–1

Vaqta, 237–8

varicella: *see* chicken pox

varicella vaccine, *see chicken pox* (varicella) vaccine

variolation, 6; definition of, 5

Varivax, 234–5

Vasotec, 208

Vella, Philip P., 162 n36

veterinary vaccines, 58, 127–32, 147; *see also* Marek's disease

Villarejos, Victor, 112, 236

virology, *see by name of disease*

Virus and Cell Biology Research, *see* Merck Virus and Cell Biology Research

vitamins: Merck production of, 38, 56, 58, 120, 124, 130

Walter Reed Army Institute of Research, 64, 66, 81, 85, 106, 153, 236; Department of Respiratory Diseases, 64–5, 70, 72–3, 74–5; Division of Communicable Diseases, 65

Walter Reed Army Medical Graduate School, 69

Walton, R., 162 n36

Washington University, 125

Weibel, Robert E., 89, 102